CHANGE

First Published in 2012
Published by Whitebeam Publishing
1 Nightingale Mews
Saffron Walden
Essex
CB10 2BQ

www.whitebeampublishing.co.uk

Designed by Paul Barrett Book Production, Cambridge www.pbbp.co.uk
Whitebeam Publishing logo designed by Joanna Whittle. Copyright © Joanna Whittle

ISBN 978-0-9571408-0-6

This book is not intended as a substitute for medical advice. The reader should consult a doctor in matters relating to his or her health and particularly with respect to any symptoms of stress or otherwise that may require medical attention.

Printed and bound by Lightning Source UK Ltd

CHANGE

Profound Changes To Transform Stress,
Fear And Self-Doubt Into
New Confidence And True Power

MAGGIE WHITTLE & SYLVIA GODDARD

WHITEBEAM PUBLISHING

Maggie's dedication with love is to John, Jo, Don, Mandy, Holly, Rowan and Stuart.

Sylvia's dedication with love is to Paul, Callum and Liam and her parents James and Margaret

Contents

Acknowledgments

We wish to express our gratitude to wonderful 'Ian Miller' for his support, humour and for the unending wisdom and generosity he has shown us.

Our special thanks go to Genevieve Miller for her good advice, kindness and willingness to offer help whenever needed.

We thank Helen Larsen for her insight and help.

Big thanks go out to John Whittle for all his sustenance, patience and good humour.

We thank Paul Goddard for his humorous creative outbursts.

Finally, we want to thank all our clients for teaching us so much, and for the brave and courageous changes they allowed us to witness.

A few words from Maggie and Sylvia

Our years of experience of helping people have let us truly see and fully understand how many people are missing out on their health, happiness and emotional development because of stress.

We have seen how so many competent and capable people have been trapped and held back in important areas of their lives because of too much stress.

We have seen how stress is implicated in most physical health problems as well as mental and emotional difficulties.

We have also seen how quickly people using our programme have turned their lives around for the better, gained a new sense of freedom and vigour and brought creative energy back into their lives.

This has driven us to share our unique programme with you. A tried and tested programme that *really* works! A programme with multiple approaches that everyone can benefit from!

We wish you well and it is our heartfelt desire that you will reap the many benefits that this book offers and build a happier, more fulfilling life for yourself.

About our powerful, unique book

This book will give you the life skills and resources to control the stress in your life.

It will also give you the life skills and resources to develop mentally, emotionally and spiritually and be your own unique, powerful, beautiful self.

You will be able to live a happier, healthier and more enjoyable life.

You will be able to get the most out of your life.

Our book is packed with brief necessary information, wisdom, illustrative scenarios, simple powerful strategies, practical skills and enjoyable, quick step-by-step techniques.

Our tools and resources are light-hearted and humorous and will enable you to make quick, positive and profound changes to your life.

They have been tried and tested and are proved to be very effective.

This is a book you can get great benefit from right away. It is a book that can benefit you throughout your whole life. It may well be the best gift you can ever give yourself.

This powerful book will give you the ability to:

- Recognise and control the stress in your life, free yourself from unnecessary worry and anxiety.
- Break free from those untrue beliefs about yourself that fill you with self-doubt and knock your confidence and self-esteem.
- Discover the truth about yourself and realise your true value and worth, your inner power, and your vast capabilities.
- Bring more sunshine into your life by adopting more helpful views and ways of dealing with life situations.
- Build up true confidence and robust self-esteem that will keep on growing.
- Improve your overall health and build a stronger immune system.

How you will benefit

- You will become more focused, calm, aware, dynamic and more competent in all areas of your life.
- You will be able to develop the confidence, capabilities and talents to have the life you want.
- You will gain excellent resources and practical life skills to enable you to advance your emotional development and emotional intelligence.
- You will find it easier to foster better relationships.
- Your emotional reactions to situations, such as being angry, distressed or anxious, will become more proportionate to what is actually happening and less subject to a stressful, anxious, often clouded, perspective.
- You will develop more courage, peace of mind and joy in your life.
- You will feel more energetic and alive and you will gain the ability to deal with life experiences in a way that works *for* you rather than against you.
- You will feel more capable of sorting out and resolving bothersome situations in your life.
- You will be able to build a happier, healthier, more fulfilling life for yourself.

This book is not intended to be read like a novel.

It is a great everyday stress-control book, an emotional and spiritual self-development book, and it is packed with life skills and resources.

For easy use, our book is divided into two parts

Both parts of our book contain extensive easy-to-use techniques, resources and life skills, backed up by many excellent scenarios and examples. As you work through *Part One*, you will see cross-references to particular Resources in *Part Two* where you will find more in-depth methods to bring about more profound changes.

Work with *Part One* and *Part Two* together

Spend some time familiarising yourself with the chapters in *Part One* and *Part Two*. *They are complementary to each other.*

For example, in *Part One* you may be gaining great skills to manage and control your stress. However, if you have difficulty and find that your self-esteem remains low, you may need to go to *Part Two* to change some *core untruths* you hold about yourself in order to build more robust self-esteem.

Part Two contains great resources on how to recognise quickly and change **four major untrue core beliefs** that promote our stress levels because they are so closely linked to our *personal power*, our *inner security*, our *capabilities* and our *self-worth*. Changing them will raise your self-esteem and confidence by a significant degree and have a wonderful positive impact on every aspect of your life.

Make this little book your friend

Let this book be with you as a friend – dipping in and out of it, choosing a bit of wisdom – a practical exercise or resource as needed.

Anytime you are stressed, pick up the book and choose an appropriate chapter and exercise from the list of chapters that will help you deal more ably with the stressful situation you are struggling with.

Some effective techniques we use

We shall use techniques that we have found from experience to be the most effective in helping people gain control over their stress and get their power and lives back.

These same techniques will be extremely effective and powerful in helping you to make essential changes quickly. As a bonus, they are very easy and uplifting to work through.

We shall describe and give you *The Most Powerful*, easy-to-use techniques used in the fields of psychology, self-development, hypnotherapy, stress management, life coaching, cognitive behavioural therapy (CBT), neuro-linguistic programming (NLP), directed imagery, metaphorical therapeutic targeted stories, and HeartMath, among others. They will enable you to relinquish those of your beliefs and patterns that promote stress and hold you back in your life.

What makes these techniques so effective?

The answer is that most of them make you use your own imagination and all major changes begin with your imagination. Without your imagination, you would be static and stuck.

Most people don't realise that we use our imagination all the time without being consciously aware of it. Even simple things like planning a meal, organising our workload, going on a journey, and figuring out how to manage various situations demand that we use our imagination.

We use our imagination when communicating with others – telling our story and experiences. We use our imagination to envisage new possibilities, to invent, design or create anything new, or even when thinking of a new way of doing something, or perhaps a day out.

The power of our imagination

Imagining is not just about being able to see pictures in your mind's eye, it includes using your five senses – what you can see or hear, touch, taste or smell – as well as being aware of your feelings and sensations.

We can all imagine a particular sound, a particular taste, a particular smell, a physical sensation in our body, a feeling or an emotion.

Whenever we imagine an experience vividly – using our senses – it is as if we were really living the experience. We actually are experiencing emotionally and physically what we are imagining. We often use our imagination to fantasise and daydream and make ourselves feel good.

Our imagination can make us stressed

Unfortunately, we often use our powerful imagination in a negative way and stress ourselves out. For example, how many times do you envisage the worst-case scenario and make yourself anxious and worried and stressed for nothing?

Such is the power of your imagination! Even small children can frighten themselves and be afraid of going to bed because they imagine monsters in the cupboard.

Some of our smart and wonderfully simple techniques will enable you to use the power of your imagination to make powerful, dramatic, positive changes to your life.

Set yourself free and live your best life!

One way or another, we are continually creating our own reality by our habitual thoughts, views, attitudes, choices and behaviours. Sometimes the reality we are creating for ourselves limits us in many ways.

Human life is about growth and change and becoming more aware and conscious so that we can choose how to live more fully. If we don't grow mentally, emotionally and spiritually, we shall stagnate and remain underdeveloped in certain areas of our lives; or we may even regress. In the end, we shall be left feeling resentful and disillusioned, having missed out in life.

Working on our personal development and growth is not a luxury, it is the most intelligent thing we can do. It is an absolute necessity for becoming our best, for living the best life we can, and for our evolution as human beings. This includes developing and balancing all aspects of our lives.

Unlike our physical growth, our personal growth and development can continue until the day we die. On those levels we really can remain forever young and free. We really do have a *lifetime* to make every effort to become better versions of ourselves. Every day we live on this earth gives us the chance to bring more such growth and development into our lives.

The biggest stumbling-blocks that hold us back are:

- Our fears and anxieties, our underlying unhelpful patterns and those beliefs and behaviours that promote our stress levels.

● Our lack of the knowledge, skills and resources needed to evolve and grow. (Never forget that our personal growth and development also involves taking care of our body.)

This book will enable you to conquer most of the anxieties and fears that promote your stress levels. It will enable you to recognise and step out of your own self-created limitations, thoughts and unhelpful behaviours.

Each step you take on your own personal self-development journey will lead to greater freedom for yourself.

Come with us, step by step, and discover your own freedom and power.

PART
ONE

1
Get To Know
All About Stress

Knowledge and insight are power!

The more knowledge and insight we have about anything that affects our life deeply, the more able we are to deal with it successfully.

This particularly applies to *Stress*. The more knowledge, understanding and insight you can gain about the *Stress in Your Life*, the more successful you will be at getting a much *Better Life for Yourself*. Not only a better life for yourself but you will take a big leap forward in your emotional development.

Cast light on this thing called stress

We are talking to you from years of experience of treating people from all walks of life suffering from stress. It doesn't matter how competent and capable you are in many aspects of your life – because you are human, you are open to stress and its harmful effects.

One of the most important things that you may ever do for yourself is to learn all about stress. You can learn how to recognise it and minimise it in your life.

Whatever your circumstances are, come along with us now, step by step, and we will show you how you can transform your life.

Who gets so stressed?

Well, you are not alone in the business of getting stressed. Everyone gets stressed; it is part of being human. Do you know that stress affects people of all ages and all walks of life? A bit of moderate, short-term stress is good for us but, sadly, prolonged high levels of stress are common and on the increase now, affecting our health and happiness.

Smart people learn all about stress

Smart people learn about stress. They know that their health and happiness depend on it. They know that no one else can take care of their health and happiness except themselves, no matter how much someone else may care about them.

You too can be equally smart and realise that you are the keeper of your health and happiness. You too can have a better life by learning all about stress now.

You have learned so many things in life – to walk, and talk, even when you were just a babe. Throughout your life, you have developed so many capabilities and resources.

By learning how to minimise stress in your life, you can create a happier, healthier and more fulfilling life for yourself. This is where your true confidence, power and happiness lie.

Significant 'stressors' are easier to recognise

Most of us can recognise those significant stressful life events such as the loss of a loved one; going through a divorce or a relationship split-up; coping with serious illness in ourselves or with someone close; or having major financial difficulties. These events are called stressors and, in the course of our lives, we shall all have to deal with many significant stressors. However distressing or upsetting, it will really make a big difference if you learn how to deal with them in the best possible way.

Minor 'stressors' can build up

Minor hassles and frustrations are part and parcel of our everyday lives.

You are probably very familiar with everyday worries and frustrations such as your car breaking down; your train being cancelled; your boiler not working; your child coming home from school and telling you he/she is being bullied; a friend letting you down; your children being more demanding and noisy; someone eating the lunch that you were keeping in the fridge. You can quickly bounce back unscathed from all these – if you know how to cope well.

Sometimes the stress and tension from all these everyday minor hassles and frustrations can mount up, and leave you feeling less able to cope with life or enjoy life.

Like most of us, you were probably never taught how to manage stress. At times, you may feel that stress is controlling you. You may get so used to feeling stressed that you accept it as being normal.

If we don't take time to relax each day to recharge our batteries, our everyday stress can insidiously build up, leaving us in a state of chronic ongoing stress.

When stress becomes ongoing – take note!

Ongoing stress, called *Chronic Stress*, is when we get into such a state that there is never any let-up.

How this affects us will depend on the intensity of this type of stress. It can be quite difficult to recognise if you are suffering from *Chronic Stress* and many people take anti-depressants or develop a physical complaint.

Many of our ongoing fears, worries and insecurities can play a big part in keeping us anxious and we can feel that there is no end to them. Have you ever felt like that?

Many situations such as heavy workloads, ongoing relationship difficulties, chronic loneliness and isolation, having trouble making ends meet, being unable to find a job and feeling disillusioned can cause this kind of ongoing stress and do not have quick solutions.

Now, add to this everyday minor hassles and we can easily be left frazzled, fatigued and worn out. We may find ourselves unable to switch off, rest or rejuvenate ourselves, or regain balance. In this state we are like a car revving at top speed with the accelerator stuck down. Our engine is working too hard and something has to give to stay in balance.

> The intensity of our stress levels, along with the length of time we remain stressed, will determine their impact on us.

Your body knows how to handle acute stress

Your body is able to cope with everyday frustrations once you know how best to approach them.

Here is a simple example of how it works. Imagine that you accidentally squirt tomato sauce down the front of your dress or white shirt just before an important meeting where you want to impress. Immediately, your **Stress Response** will kick in to give you a boost of energy and focus to help you adapt to the tomato sauce spill and deal with it. If you deal with the situation in a helpful way, your body will soon relax and go back into balance. Now if you don't manage the stress induced by this minor event you may continue to worry and beat yourself up over the spill and then you will remain stressed for a much longer time.

Moderate short-term stress can be good for you

Short-term moderate stress, called *Optimal Stress*, is good for you and for a healthy, balanced life. This moderate stress gives you a quick boost of adrenaline and enables you to rise to the challenges in your daily life and perform at your best.

By giving you more energy, clarity, focus and motivation, you can **master new skills** and perform better under pressure.

Optimal Stress can inspire and stimulate you to explore new possibilities and find good solutions. Besides, you need a certain amount of this type of stress to enjoy life – to spice it up and give you more excitement and passion. The right amount of *Optimal Stress* can have a positive effect on your body.

Your everyday performance is related to your overall stress levels. Too much stress and you can become distressed and anxious and your performance goes down. Too much relaxation and you can become lethargic and dopy. It really is all about having the right balance of stress (*optimal stress*) for you to perform at your best.

Prolonged stress can damage your health

We want you to know that prolonged stress can damage your physical health and create mental and emotional problems.

Be aware that up to 80—90 per cent of physical and emotional ailments are stress-related, induced by stress and maintained or made worse by stress.

Stress and depression are closely linked and can feed off each other.

Prolonged stress can break down your immune system, which is your body's natural defence against illness and disease.

The chemical and hormonal changes that go with chronic stress can have a damaging effect on every single organ of your body.

Prolonged stress can make you grow older and sadder more quickly. You deserve to be healthy, beautiful and young at heart – whatever your age.

And here is the great news! When you control your stress, you definitely get on top of your worries and anxieties and bring more confidence, joy and happiness into your life.

Take heart, we are all in this together

This book will give you the information and tools not only to relieve your stress but to improve every aspect of your health, including building up your magical, powerful immune system.

This book has the power to rejuvenate your life, give you super-confidence and greatly increase your self-esteem and personal power.

Always know that, with the right knowledge and tools, you are your own greatest healer.

2
Our Emergency Stress Response

What happens when our stress response is triggered?

We all have a stress response – also known as the *Fight or Flight* response. This is our body's primitive, automatic, emergency response. It is our most basic survival strategy, which is genetically hard-wired into our brain. It gets turned on when we feel under threat of a physical attack. Our whole system goes on high alert and we get a tremendous boost of energy and strength to fight for our life or run away to safety, hence the term *Fight or Flight*.

Once you had dealt with the enemy, fought or run to safety, your body would have discharged the high energy and gone back into balance. This *Fight or Flight* is still very relevant today if your life is in physical danger – it can, in fact, save your life.

When our 'fight or flight' is turned on our body gets very busy

As soon as our *Fight or Flight* is turned on, a specific part of our nervous system (referred to as the sympathetic nervous system) gets activated and powerful stress hormones like adrenaline and cortisol are released into our blood. This gives us the strength and ability to deal with the threat. These powerful hormones cause dramatic changes in all the major systems of the body. We really get ready for battle.

Know what happens in your body when your 'stress response' is turned on

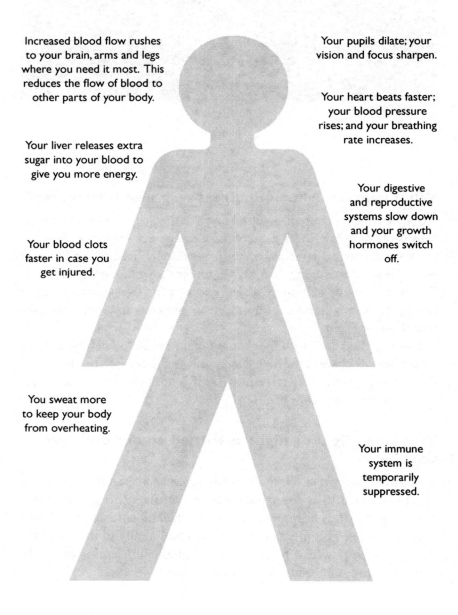

Increased blood flow rushes to your brain, arms and legs where you need it most. This reduces the flow of blood to other parts of your body.

Your pupils dilate; your vision and focus sharpen.

Your heart beats faster; your blood pressure rises; and your breathing rate increases.

Your liver releases extra sugar into your blood to give you more energy.

Your digestive and reproductive systems slow down and your growth hormones switch off.

Your blood clots faster in case you get injured.

You sweat more to keep your body from overheating.

Your immune system is temporarily suppressed.

Long-term, this situation would not be good for your health

Our stress response has now gone a bit haywire

1 Our **Stress Response** gets triggered not only when we are in physical danger but in everyday situations that frustrate or put extra pressure on us (our stressors). So, basically it fails to distinguish between our everyday stressors and life-threatening emergencies. This can be a major problem because every time our **Stress Response** is switched on powerful stress hormones flood our body.

2 Our brain can also activate our **Stress Response** just by *perceiving* a threat. This is because the primitive part of the brain is unable to detect whether a threat is a *real* one or just an *imagined* one. Many of our fears are unfounded, yet they can create untold stress in us.

3 Whenever our brain registers anything that it *perceives* as a threat to our emotional security or our ego – be that internal worry or anger, or something as simple as having an argument or being embarrassed – it can turn on our **Stress Response** and flood our body with stress hormones. That is why our *ongoing* thoughts of doubt, uncertainty and worry will keep turning on our **Stress Response**.

4 The *ongoing* pressures on many people from poverty, social deprivation, lack of education, lack of opportunities and extreme inequality can also keep those affected in a state of constant insecurity and so in chronic stress.

The degree of the threat we feel in any situation will determine the strength of our Stress Response.

Do some people get more stressed than others?

Yes, they do indeed – some people have a much easier life than others and have fewer stressors to cope with. However, there are some life events and situations that will stress anyone.

Some people handle stress better than others. Some people have an inherited disposition to worry and fret more easily. Anyone who has experienced a traumatic childhood may be more easily stressed (and that includes long-term being bullied when young).

Our beliefs and attitudes

Our underlying beliefs, thoughts and attitudes determine how we react to life experiences and how we respond to pressure. So they play a big part in determining our stress levels.

Don't worry – you can turn off your **Stress Response** right away and give yourself a break.

This is your golden ticket to make a happier life for yourself!

How to switch off your stress response

Specific breathing techniques will instantly switch off your Stress Response and bring relaxing hormones into your blood.

The following two breathing exercises will quickly relax you. It really is more than worthwhile to learn them.

In both these exercises it is vital that you make your **out breath** (exhalation) longer than your **in breath** (inhalation).

Prolonging your out breath stimulates your relaxation response and that is why it is so vital to make sure your out breath is longer than your in breath in both these exercises.

Exercise 1   Calm breath

Sit down. Gently close your eyes.

1 Breathe out slowly through your mouth, emptying your belly of air.

2 Now take in a short breath from your belly, inhaling through your nose **to the count of 5** (do not pause between numbers – just count as you would normally do).

3 Immediately breathe out slowly through pursed lips, emptying your belly completely **to the count of 9** (as if you were slowly letting the air out of a balloon).

4 Continue with this pattern of breathing for a few minutes.

5 Open your eyes and feel good.

The 'Sigh Breath' will enable you to release some tension from your body and bring relaxing hormones into your blood.

Initially, a few Sigh Breaths about every hour or so will halt the build-up of tension in your body.

Exercise 2   Sigh breath

Sit down for a few moments.

1 Take a short breath in through your nose.

2 Without pausing, **Blow your breath out very slowly for as long as you can** until there is no more breath left in you. Your out breath is akin to a long slow sigh.
As you sigh, release as much physical tension as you can from your body. Let your shoulders drop down and back, let your jaw open and relax, and as you let your body relax, say the words 'calm and relaxed'.

You can do either of these exercises whenever you feel tense or stressed. You can do them anywhere, anytime – you don't even need to sit down to do them.

Getting to know the everyday situations and worrying thoughts that trigger your Stress Response is the first major step towards learning to control your stress.

Each time you become aware of these triggers, pause and take a few relaxing breaths.

Important reminder No. 1
Turn off your **Stress Response** quickly by relaxing breathing.

3
How To Recognise
Stress In Yourself

How stress can show up in your body

Become familiar with how stress can affect your body. This knowledge will give you the power to take quick, positive action as needs be.

The specific effects of stress on us will vary from person to person. Some people experience more of the *physical* signs of stress in their body than others. Some will experience more in their *thought patterns*; others more on the *emotional level*; while in others it may be more evident in their *behaviour*.

Since most of our stress is not caused by physical danger, we are often unable to fight or run to discharge the tension. It builds up in our body, stressing our organs if we don't deliberately discharge it through exercise or some other physical activity for instance.

Have a look at the diagram on the next page to see how stress can affect your body.

Recognise any of these common symptoms of stress in your body? Don't expect to have all of them!

Do you get frequent headaches or feel light-headed or dizzy?

Do you frequently get a dry mouth or mouth ulcers?

Do you suffer from pains in your neck or back? Or muscle spasms or cramps?

Do you frequently get butterflies in your stomach, bloating, burping or cramps?

Do you often feel cold, clammy, sweaty or shaky?

Do you have any persistent nervous habits like fidgeting, foot-tapping, trembling or twitching?

Do you clench your jaw or grind your teeth at night?

Do you hold your breath at times or breathe faster or often sigh?

Do you get a faster heartbeat or tightness in your chest?

Do you often get constipation or diarrhoea or both? Do you have frequent urination?

Is your sexual function impaired in any way?

Do you frequently get itching, rashes, hives, or goose pimples?

Do you have any sleep problems?

Now, check out your body for any tension

- Sit where you are without altering your normal position in any way.
- Note your posture. How are you sitting? Are your shoulders hunched or relaxed? Is your back slouched?
- Can you feel tightness, pain or discomfort in your head, any tightness or spasm in your jaw?
- Do you notice any tension in your neck, including the back of your neck? Do you notice any tension in your shoulders or back?
- Do you notice any tension, pain or discomfort around your rib cage?
- Or any tension or knot in your stomach?
- What about the muscles in your buttocks, thighs, calves and ankles – any tension there?
- Do you have any tension or pain in your elbows, arms or hands, ankles or feet?

For the time being, just take note of any areas in your body that feel tense.

Now try Exercise 1 and release some of your tension.

Exercise 1   Squeeze and Let Go will allow you to release body tension.

Familiarise yourself with this exercise and then begin:

- Take a normal breath (do not breathe in deeply).
- Hold your breath and at the same time begin to clench every muscle in your body. Clench only as tightly as is comfortable for you – for a few seconds perhaps.
- Squeeze your eyes closed and clench your jaw shut – but not too tightly.
- Clench your fists, hunch your shoulders and clench all your upper body muscles.
- Press your feet into the floor, curl your toes, and clench your thighs and buttocks.
- Squeeze in your abdomen.
- Hold your body clenched for a few moments.
- Then breathe out slowly with a whoosh ……….. and slowly release every clenched muscle in your body.

- Shake your body a bit — do a body wobble — legs, arms, hands.
- Feel your body go all floppy and relaxed.
- Take a big stretch and then move your body around for a few moments.

Throughout the day you can treat yourself to this little gem anywhere, anytime.

Stress can affect your thoughts and emotions

Changes and challenges in life are inevitable and help us develop as human beings. How boring life would be without them. Anything that puts too high demands on us or forces us to change can be stressful. Even positive events such as getting married, moving to a new place, leaving home, buying a house, can be a bit stressful for many, yet exciting at the same time and there's nothing wrong with that!

However, if life's challenges and changes make us feel overwhelmed, we can react by feeling out of control, anxious and fearful.

As stress can affect our mental and emotional equilibrium and our behaviour, check out the next two diagrams to note the changes that can occur.

Recognise any of these common symptoms in yourself?

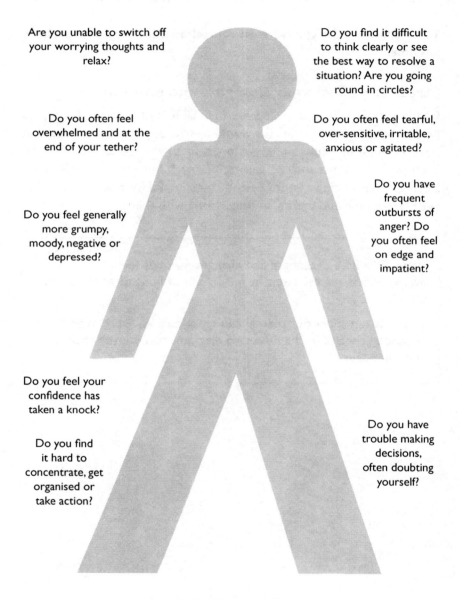

Are you unable to switch off your worrying thoughts and relax?

Do you often feel overwhelmed and at the end of your tether?

Do you feel generally more grumpy, moody, negative or depressed?

Do you feel your confidence has taken a knock?

Do you find it hard to concentrate, get organised or take action?

Do you find it difficult to think clearly or see the best way to resolve a situation? Are you going round in circles?

Do you often feel tearful, over-sensitive, irritable, anxious or agitated?

Do you have frequent outbursts of anger? Do you often feel on edge and impatient?

Do you have trouble making decisions, often doubting yourself?

Do you find it hard to see the funny side of life? Have you lost your perspective on life?

Some of our unhelpful behaviour when under stress – check it out!

Avoid sorting important things out?

Not bothering to eat properly?

Procrastinate and avoid responsibilities?

'Comfort eat' or turn to drugs or alcohol?

Overwork?

Hide away from our problems and difficulties – avoid even talking about them?

Be irritable and snappy and appear unreasonable?

Avoid people, avoid socialising and become isolated?

Neglect ourselves and our own needs?

Buy far more than is necessary and/or over-exercise?

Neglect those close to us, e.g. partner, children?

Pick arguments or fights with people and be unreasonable?

4
Breathe Better And Stress Less

Our breathing and stress connection

Ongoing stress and poor breathing habits are often linked. Have you ever felt a bit short of air – like a fish out of water? If you do, maybe you need to look a little closer at your breathing pattern.

Have you ever noticed that, when you get stressed, you tend to breathe faster and shallower? If you have *prolonged (chronic)* stress, you may get stuck in this pattern of fast upper chest breathing or an irregular breathing pattern. This over-breathing pattern is known as *chronic hyperventilation.*

Stress can be kept in place by the way we breathe

The way you breathe really matters when it comes to controlling your stress levels.

With an over-breathing pattern, your heart will have to beat faster to supply enough blood and nutrients to your body. This in turn can trigger your stress response.

There is nothing more important in your life than breathing – *breathing is life.*

If you have a pattern of *chronic hyperventilation*, good breathing habits will need to be relearned and practised. If not, you will keep yourself in a stressed state and gasp like the fish out of water!

Over-breathing is a lot more common than you think. We noticed how common this pattern was in many people with chronic stress.

Prolonged stress can reset your breathing pattern

For some people, even after the prolonged stressful situation has passed, an over-breathing pattern may continue. One reason may be that the breathing centre in the brain may have reset itself at a faster pace.

Chronic hyperventilation and chronic stress seem to feed off each other and form a vicious cycle. Chronic stress can perpetuate this over-breathing pattern which, in turn, keeps activating your stress response.

You can easily learn how to change this pattern and you will be amazed at the positive effect on your life. Breathing is life's most precious gift and it is free!

Important – a delicate balance of oxygen and carbon dioxide

A healthy breathing pattern is necessary to maintain the right balance of oxygen and carbon dioxide levels for our body to function properly. The right balance of carbon dioxide is necessary to carry sufficient oxygen from the blood to the brain, vital organs and tissues.

Chronic hyperventilation causes a decrease in carbon dioxide levels in our blood, resulting in a shortage of vital oxygen. When this happens, the body signals a need for more oxygen and there is a tendency to breathe faster in an effort to get more oxygen. Then we do the very opposite of what would help. We take in *even more* oxygen (by breathing in faster) which we are *unable to use* and so deplete our vital carbon dioxide levels even further. Isn't it ironic that we can take in too much oxygen and be unable to use it?

If you have a pattern of upper chest breathing, you need to breathe in *less oxygen* and allow *carbon dioxide* to build up a little. Do this by using your 5 to 9 breathing pattern as in Exercise 1, Calm Breath, page 10.

This will stimulate your relaxation response and bring relaxing hormones into your body, lessening your tension.

Although chronic stress is the most common cause of *chronic hyperventilation*, it may be caused by poor posture, such as sitting hunched up in front of a computer all day, or by a medical condition. It is always best to be checked by your doctor.

Look out for your body's clues

- You can have this damaging breathing pattern for years without knowing it.
- You may find yourself frequently sighing or yawning, or holding your breath, or feeling a bit short of breath.
- You may feel a little light-headed or dizzy or experience a foggy, unreal sensation at times.
- You may have a feeling of impending panic (a very high percentage of panic attacks are due to chronic hyperventilation).
- You may feel sweaty, a bit shaky and clammy at times. Your stomach may feel bloated and you may belch a lot from swallowing too much air.
- This shortage of carbon dioxide can cause cramps and a narrowing of the blood vessels giving rise to muscle spasms, tingling or numbness in different parts of your body.
- You may have various muscular aches and pains, especially in the neck, the back and the shoulders.

The long-term imbalance of oxygen and carbon dioxide levels can damage your physical health. It can make you exhausted, weaken your immune system and open you up to serious illness.

It can make you feel miserable. It can make you feel irritable, grumpy, on edge, tearful, anxious, fearful and even paranoid or depressed.

Now you know about this thing called *chronic hyperventilation*. You have learned how you can contribute to this pattern by taking in *too much oxygen* and reducing adequate carbon dioxide levels.

You can turn this around by regularly practising your relaxing breathing techniques and re-establishing good breathing patterns.

Exercise I   De-stress and relax by using your breath

You can switch off your emergency stress response button and maintain adequate carbon dioxide levels which will allow you to use your vital oxygen efficiently and bring calming hormones into your blood.

This exercise is quite similar to the exercise you learned in Chapter 3 except that it uses the power of your imagination to help you relax even more.

Use this exercise whenever you feel yourself getting stressed, have an upcoming event that you are worried about, or just whenever you want to relax.

Do this exercise at least 3–4 times a day for a few minutes – it will help to reset your brain to a healthier pattern of breathing.

Remember that it is vital you make your out breath (exhalation) longer than your in breath (inhalation).

1 Gently close your eyes if appropriate.
2 Breathe out slowly through your mouth, emptying your belly of air.
3 Now take in a short breath from your belly, inhaling through your nose to **the count of 5,** (just count as you normally would). Imagine that you are breathing in **calming blue light.**
4 Immediately breathe out slowly through pursed lips, emptying your belly completely **to the count of 9** (as if you were slowly letting the air out of a balloon). As you breathe out, imagine the tension leaving your body like **black smoke.**
5 Continue with this pattern of breathing for a few minutes.
6 Open your eyes and feel good and relaxed.

> Regular exercise will also improve your breathing pattern, release body tension and reduce your stress levels.

You are probably aware that regular exercise such as walking, swimming, running, cycling and sports are all very beneficial to your health.

However, even something as short and simple as 10 minutes' marching on the spot with your arms swinging; going for a brisk walk around the block; or dancing around to music you like will also have a positive impact on your health and your breathing. It's a good place to start and build on.

Good posture can help you breathe better and stress less

Now is a good time for you to look at your posture and improve it if needed. It will go a long way to helping you release tension and stress.

> Poor posture can hamper your breathing and contribute to your stress.
>
> The muscle tension and slumping of poor posture can impede our breathing.
>
> It can make us breathe shallower and faster.
>
> This itself triggers our stress reaction and maintains it until we change our posture.

Poor posture is common nowadays due to our lifestyle and sitting for long periods of time, often at a computer. Our bodies were designed to move and be more active.

Do you know that your posture also plays a major role in how you feel? The close interaction between our body, mind and emotions means that poor posture and slumping send a message to your subconscious mind, creating a 'down mood' for you.

When you are feeling relaxed and confident, your posture will visibly reflect this. Assuming a confident, relaxed posture, even if we don't always feel it, can also be helpful. So throughout your day be aware of your posture and correct it if necessary.

It is important to move around and stretch frequently throughout your day and try to fit in some short exercise every day.

Important reminder No. 1
Take note of your breathing when you feel stressed and switch off your stress response immediately.

Important reminder No. 2
A little bit of exercise is a good place to start!

Important reminder No. 3
Keep an eye on your posture.

5
Find A Retreat
Of Your Own

Switch off now and relax

You deserve a real break. You need a special time when you can switch off, relax and be yourself. Set aside 10–15 minutes a day just for yourself.

Create your own *Peaceful Haven* – a place where you can find peace and where fluster and worry begin to fade away.

The benefits of doing this exercise are invaluable. If done regularly, it will reduce accumulative stress, anxiety and worry. It will relieve some of the physical symptoms of stress and create a more positive, hopeful attitude. Your clarity and concentration will improve. It definitely will give your confidence and self-worth a well-deserved boost.

In this exercise we shall show you how to direct your imagination towards bringing deep relaxation and balance to your mind and body. It is easy to learn and well worth the effort.

It is a truly transformative, enjoyable exercise that you can use throughout your whole life.

How does it work?

Your unconscious mind really cannot differentiate between what is a *real* experience and what is an *imagined* one. Therefore, whenever we imagine an event vividly, we *actually* experience emotionally and physically what we are imagining. Chemical changes in our body reflect this.

By just imagining yourself relaxing in a very calm, peaceful scene, pleasurable to your senses, you will bring relaxing hormones into your blood, release stress and tension from your body, and eventually feel genuinely calm and peaceful.

Instructions for creating your peaceful haven

This is just one example of how to create your own *peaceful haven*. You may prefer to create your own in any setting of your choice.

To get the most out of this exercise, read it through a few times to become familiar with it.

Sit or lie down in a comfortable place where you won't be disturbed for 10–15 minutes.

- Close your eyes.
- Do your relaxing breathing (see Exercise 1, Calm Breath, page 10) for a few moments.
- Imagine yourself walking down 5 steps leading to a beautiful blue and gold door that has your name on it.
- Nobody else can see this door but you. It is your door to your own secret, peaceful garden – your safe haven.

- To enter this garden, all you need to do is imagine touching the door. It opens, you go through, and it closes behind you.
- You can go in and out of this door any time you want by just imagining it. Nobody else can enter unless invited.

- Imagine now that you are in your peaceful garden – your safe haven, where you can relax and be at ease.
- Your garden is very secluded with high walls covered in grasses and moss and beautiful red, yellow, pink, blue and orange flowers.
- You stand still for a moment in your garden and sense how peaceful, how quiet, how calm it is here.
- As you breathe in, imagine you are breathing the stillness and calm into your body, mind and spirit. Note how your body is beginning to relax and the tension starting to ebb away.
- You begin to feel a great sense of peace and calmness spreading through your mind and emotions.

- You look up at the sky and it is bright blue without a single cloud.
- There is a patch of wild meadow flowers to the right of where you are standing. Their scent is so soothing. You touch the delicate petals of a red poppy and feel its soft silkiness beneath your fingers.
- A soothing, gentle, warm breeze touches your face, bringing welcome comfort.
- You can feel the warmth of the sunshine on your skin and this makes you feel even more comfortable, relaxed and at ease.

- You walk barefoot along the grassy path and feel the warmth of the springy soft grass beneath your feet.
- You feel a sense of belonging and closeness to the earth.
- You come to a beautiful small waterfall that is tumbling gently over the garden wall.
- You sit on a big flat, smooth, white stone and you listen to the tinkling and soft splashes as the water falls into a small, crystal-clear pool close by. You take a handful of water and taste its cool fresh cleanness.

- You notice a big, white, soft fluffy, relaxing chair close by.
- You go over and sink down into it, feeling your whole body relaxing, cocooned in its fluffy softness.
- You feel an overwhelming sense of peace.
- Now just let yourself be lulled by the gentle soft tinkling sound of your waterfall.
- Relax … enjoy … be still … relax … feel at peace …
- Say aloud to yourself 'My Peaceful Haven'.

When you want to come back to reality, tell yourself that you will count from 1 to 5 and, when you reach 5, you will be fully present and energised.

Try to do this exercise a few times a week.

The more you do it, the better you will train yourself to relax quickly and enjoy more benefit.

You can go to your *peaceful haven* at any time. If you can't sleep, it's a great place to go.

This is not just a powerful tool for stress management but an important life skill that can be used any time you need that peaceful break.

You can re-experience the tranquillity of your peaceful haven at any time

Whenever you feel overwrought and need a few moments' peace, sit down where you are safe and comfortable and won't be disturbed:

● Take a few relaxing breaths.

● Just imagine yourself again in your Peaceful Haven, sitting on your big, white, soft fluffy chair, lulled by the gentle tinkling soft sound of your waterfall, and say silently to yourself 'My Peaceful Haven' and you will rapidly bring yourself into a peaceful state of mind.

● When you want to be fully alert, just tell yourself that you will count from 1 to 5 and, when you reach 5, you will be fully alert.

6a
Are You Really Under Threat?

Is your imagination tricking you?

Do you know that most of our everyday stress is really an invention of our imagination? 'Really?' you may be asking yourself. This invention is often based on how we *view* the situation and our *perception* of what we believe is happening. Well, get this – our *views* and *perceptions* of situations that stress us are *not always* based on truth. Rather, they are based on what we imagine to be the truth.

How can this happen to us?

Our underlying unconscious beliefs and attitudes operate outside of our conscious awareness.

They influence the way in which we view, interpret and react to each experience we encounter.

Many of our beliefs that make us stressed are outdated and not based on truth.

They were created when we were children and our understanding was limited.

(In Part Two we tell you more about how to recognise these beliefs and change them.)

Each one of us has our own beliefs and attitudes. Now you can see why some people get much more stressed than others and why some people have more confidence than others. And why some people have less confidence than others.

Let's look at the following scenario, which portrays how our perception and the meaning we give to experiences affects our stress levels.

The Mark and Paul scenario

Mark and Paul work for the same company. They live in different areas and are both stuck in a long, unexpected traffic jam. Neither of them is aware that the other one is stuck in the same traffic jam. Both men are due at the same management meeting. They both left home with plenty of time to get there.

Let's look at Paul's view and perception of what is happening

Paul does not see the traffic jam as a threat. His stress response does not get activated.

Paul feels a little disappointed but not significantly stressed

His rational, rather than his primitive, brain is in control and tells him, 'This traffic jam was totally unpredictable.'

Paul's thoughts about the situation (reflecting his unconscious beliefs)

'It's not the end of the world. I gave myself plenty of time to get there, making allowance for some delays. I have travelled here every morning for over a year and have never seen anything like this. There is not much I can do now so there is no point in worrying about it. I will get feedback from my colleagues and I will set up another meeting with the director and others involved.'

Emotionally Paul feels at ease now with the situation; he is not stressed about it.

Paul behaves in a responsible way

He takes positive action. He rings a work colleague, explaining the situation, and asks her to pass his apologies to the director and his colleagues. He picks his favourite CD and enjoys it while waiting in the traffic jam.

Now, let's look at Mark's view and perception of what is happening
He sees the situation as a total disaster. His stress response is switched on and he becomes stressed and upset. Rational thinking goes out of the window.

Emotionally Mark feels distressed, frustrated, anxious, guilty, irritable, angry and stressed out. His confidence takes a knock.

Mark's thoughts about the situation (reflecting his unconscious beliefs)
He talks to himself in an entirely negative way.

'The director and the others will be really angry with me. They will think I am incompetent for not getting there on time. I won't have my say at the meeting and I might never get the chance again. They may allocate my project to someone else. This will be a black mark against me. They will think the job is not that important to me.'

Mark then launches into some serious self-criticism
'I'm such an idiot. I am so stupid. I should have set off earlier. I can never get everything right. I am such an idiot. This couldn't happen to anyone else but me. I hate myself for being so stupid.'

He thinks he should phone and tell the office that he is stuck in a traffic jam. Then he thinks, 'Oh, no. They will think that is a pathetic excuse and they will laugh at me.' He is confused now and can't decide what to do. This makes matters worse.

The stress takes its toll on Mark physically
Since powerful stress hormones are now flooding his blood-stream, he starts to feel tension in his neck and shoulders. He gets butterflies in his stomach and feels a bit queasy. He begins to get sweaty and feels a headache coming on.

Mark's behaviour – He avoids dealing with the situation
Mark chooses the unhelpful behaviour of avoidance and doesn't ring. Nothing can be resolved now. This causes his stress levels to rise further.

When he reaches his office, Mark appears unfriendly, agitated, grumpy and a bit paranoid because he is so stressed. This makes his colleagues reluctant to engage with him.

His whole day is plagued by negative thoughts, guilt and self-doubt.

Let's take a closer look at Mark's stress reaction to the traffic jam
Mark's primitive brain saw this as a threat and instantly activated his stress response in order that he could fight or run. However, there was no one to fight and nowhere to run.

This put Mark at the mercy of his emotions and he impulsively reacted to the situation rather than consciously weighing up the type of reaction it warranted. This impulsive reaction is often called a 'knee-jerk' reaction, when our emotions take control of us rather than the other way around.

Has this ever happened to you? It happens to most of us. However, if it happens too frequently, it will end up sabotaging your life.

Mark's knee-jerk emotional reaction – why?
Like all of us, Mark's brain remembers all his past negative experiences, his emotional reactions to them and how he dealt with them. Mark's brain will use this imprinted information as a blueprint for reacting to, and dealing with, similar type situations.

Therefore, any event in the present that evokes his memories of past similar type negative experiences can trigger his stress response and the same emotional reactions and behaviours.

This reaction of fear is so immediate and happens so quickly that the rational, more sophisticated, part of the brain does not get a chance to assess the situation.

As a result, in this traffic jam, Mark finds himself in a position of intense stress where rational thinking has gone out of the window.

It would be very difficult for Mark to change his perception or look at the traffic jam from a different viewpoint with his stress response switched on. You try frying fish if your chip pan is on fire!

You need to become aware of your 'knee-jerk' stress reactions and what triggers them.

You now have a better idea of how stress can affect your thoughts, emotions and body and how that stops you getting a situation into perspective.

Important reminder No. 1
Our stress reaction will depend on how we view and interpret each situation.

Important reminder No. 2
Just because we have fearful feelings, it does not always mean that they are based on truth or reality (as you see from Mark's case).

In Chapter 6b you will learn what Mark can do to avoid a knee-jerk reaction and prevent him from getting into this highly stressed state.

6b
Stop Stressing Yourself

Stop stressing yourself like Mark!

Mark was capable – stress got the better of him

- No matter how capable you are, you too can get stressed – don't let stress get the better of you!
- When Mark felt his initial fear, his stress response was instantly switched on. Mark needed to switch off his stress response quickly by doing a few slow, relaxing breaths. This would have helped him to be more rational.
- Mark needed to remind himself that, just because he had negative thoughts, worries and feelings about his situation, his colleagues and manager, it did not mean that they were true.
- Mark needed to look at what evidence he had to support his view of the situation, his colleagues and manager. He would soon have realised that there was no evidence to back up his views. He needed to take a more optimistic approach towards the situation.
- Mark needed to talk more kindly to himself and reassure himself that he was doing his best, rather than intensifying his stress by putting himself down.
- Mark would then have had a much better chance of taking good action to deal with the situation, as Paul had done.
- In **refusing** to take action, Mark chose the worst option to further his stress. He needed to inform his work colleagues of the traffic jam and offer his apologies regarding the meeting. He also needed to get information from his colleagues about the meeting he missed – he **avoided** doing that.

To turn an everyday stressful situation into not such a big deal, try looking at it from a more realistic viewpoint.

Make yourself feel better, not worse!

The worst thing we can do in any stressful situation is to avoid dealing with it.

This increases our stress levels and decreases our confidence.

We shall get stuck with our stressful situation and take it to bed with us!

We need to face our problems and difficulties and resolve them as best we can. This will automatically make us feel better. If the outcome is not what we want, we need to accept that things don't always go to plan and we shall feel better for trying.

Paul reacted well to the traffic jam situation – but his reaction to another situation might be similar to Mark's. We all have our own faulty unconscious programmes that can easily be activated when the right button is pushed.

A good trick to gain perspective

In any stressful situation ask yourself, how much stress does this situation warrant on a scale of 1 to 10 (10 being the highest). 10 would only apply if your life were under threat.

Mostly, we exaggerate the threat and flip the number on our scale up to 8 or 9 when it should only warrant 1 or 2 or 3 and we make ourselves unduly stressed.

Look at the example sliding scale on the next page. In your imagination you can adjust your scale to reflect the level of threat to you in any stressful situation. This will put your stressor in perspective. You will be very surprised at the results; they will make you smile at yourself.

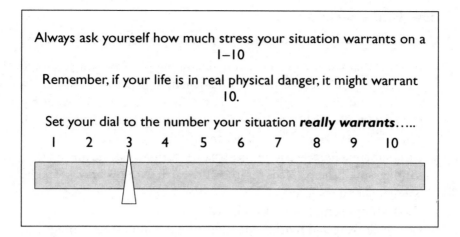

Always ask yourself how much stress your situation warrants on a 1–10

Remember, if your life is in real physical danger, it might warrant 10.

Set your dial to the number your situation **really warrants**......

Great stress-releasing exercise

Many people have found the following exercise extremely helpful in reducing their stress and worry regarding specific situations in the past, present or future (providing your life is not really under threat).

You can use it, for example, if you are anxious about having to confront someone, or deal with someone you find difficult, or you are facing the prospect of an interview, an exam, the dentist. You name it, people have found that this exercise works really well.

By creating a threatening image to represent your specific fear/anxiety and changing it into a harmless image, you will greatly reduce your anxiety.

Your unconscious mind gets the message from this imagery that the situation is not a great threat to you and you will automatically feel less anxious or fearful about it.

Read through the Bull exercise to familiarise yourself with it. Before you start, take a few relaxing breaths and close your eyes.

The Bull exercise

Create a big black fearsome bull to represent your specific fear/worry.

- Imagine that you are in a field and, separating you from the fearsome bull, is a big wall of transparent, toughened, impenetrable plastic.
- Imagine that this black bull is at least 6 foot tall. He has a great big muscular body with big, powerful, long, sharp horns that point in your direction. His eyes are large, angry-looking and red.
- He is snorting fiercely and his nostrils are flaring, with steam and snot coming out of them. He is scraping the earth with his hooves and he is agitated and restless.
- He is whipping his tail back and forth.
- He is bellowing and roaring so loudly that it is almost deafening.

Maybe you feel a little anxious at this stage. Remember now that you are in charge of this bull image.

Imagine that you have a small button in the palm of your right hand which you can press to change the bull.

- Press the button slightly and see this big black fearsome bull begin to shrink down a little. Shrink him down by a foot or two to begin with.
- Watch his tail gradually moving less and less until it is no longer whipping. Notice that he is no longer bellowing but gently moaning.
- Then shrink him down a little further.
- Watch his eyes and notice how they are returning to normal as he looks at you.
- Then shrink him down another little bit.
- He is just shaking his head in bewilderment.
- Notice now that his horns are no longer there.

- **Now notice that you are feeling a little calmer and now …..**

- Continue to press the button and shrink the bull down further until he is the size of a lamb – shrink him even smaller if you wish, even to 6 inches.
- Imagine going into the field where he is – on the other side of the toughened plastic.
- See how harmless he is – he is only a little fellow.
- Notice how smooth and shiny his black coat is.

- **You say hello to him and tell him that he is free to go as he pleases.**

- Watch him run away over the fields.

Now, notice that you are feeling less anxious about your problem.

Repeat this exercise several times for a long-standing worry and fear.

Important reminder No. 1
Every time you encounter an experience or a person that distresses you, turn off your stress response by doing relaxing breathing (see page 10). This will calm you down and provide your brain with enough oxygen for you to think more clearly and creatively.

Important reminder No. 2
Just because you have fear-based thoughts and upsetting emotions doesn't mean that they are based on reality.

Important reminder No. 3
Your perception of any experience will determine whether you are stressed by it or not. Remember to set your scale realistically.

Important reminder No. 4
By selecting an image to represent your specific worry/fear and changing it into a harmless image (as above), you will feel less worried/fearful. Repeat this exercise as often as is needed to quell your specific worry/fear.

In our next chapter you will see how a more optimistic attitude can help us cope with challenging situations in a more helpful and confident way. Also, in Resource 7, you will find a Neuro Linguistic Programming (NLP) exercise to reduce fears and worries.

7
Create A More Optimistic Attitude

Keep the sunshine in your life!

You were born with joy in your heart! Ongoing stress can make us feel negative and think in a pessimistic way. We can get stuck in this way of thinking without even being aware that it is happening to us.

Everyone thinks negatively at times. We would be very annoying if we were upbeat and happy all the time. There is nothing wrong with having a good moan and feeling sorry for ourselves – sometimes we need to do that.

If we cling to a negative outlook and attitude, we do ourselves a great disservice.

This way of thinking can even make us feel anxious and depressed, cynical and resentful.

It can keep stress hormones in our blood, creating damage.

A more optimistic view will help

When you think in a more hopeful way, most things in your life will not feel so big or daunting to you. You will feel more optimistic, your heart will be lighter, and you will be better able to handle pressure. Also, other people will like to be around you more.

A more optimistic attitude does not mean that you bury your head in the sand. It means that you face life's ups and downs, and take good action when you need to – dealing with things in a helpful way without letting them fester, learning from mistakes, changing what you can, and accepting what you can't change right away. Most of all, don't take yourself, others or life events too seriously.

A more hopeful attitude – a more positive reality for you

A more hopeful attitude, along with a more positive way of viewing situations, people and life, will create a more positive reality for you. It is important to take charge of your thoughts and learn to think in a more optimistic way so that you can get the very best out of your life.

A more positive attitude will help you be more confident and find new creative opportunities for yourself and new creative solutions for your problems.

Metaphorical imagery – to promote more optimism

Familiarise yourself with this exercise first and repeat it as often as you need to.

Sit down and take a few relaxing breaths ......

- Imagine that you are wearing a big pair of black-rimmed glasses. You are unaware that the lenses in these glasses are a dull, greyish, murky brown. Everything around you looks dull and murky – your home – the skies – the trees – the flowers – the garden – the food you eat – even the people you see around you. You yourself feel dull, unhappy and lustreless.
- An old record plays in the background – a mournful irritating dirge – that appears stuck and plays the same thing over and over.
- Somehow, you become aware that you are wearing heavy glasses and you whip them off. You throw away your glasses. You throw out the faulty stuck record.
- To your amazement, most things around you are bright, colourful and cheerful – the sun is shining, you hear birds singing, you see butterflies dancing past, the earth is alive and humming. You begin to laugh – your heart feels happy.

Important reminder No. 1
An unhealthy negative attitude will make you more stressed and unhappy.

Important reminder No. 2
Developing a more optimistic attitude will create a more positive reality for you.

8
Listen To The Wisdom Of Your Body

Have a break when your body tells you

If we follow our body's natural cycles throughout the day, we shall develop a much calmer state of mind.

Sometimes we may forgo calm, relaxing and rejuvenating times for ourselves. Taking time to relax and recharge our batteries is not a luxury; it is absolutely essential for maintaining our health, our happiness and our sanity.

It is really important that we recognise, manage and minimise the minor stressors in our life. Otherwise we may find ourselves being irritable and snappy, feeling harassed and worn out. This will make bigger stressors seem even more daunting to deal with.

Listen to your body

Research indicates that the body has its own natural energy cycle, known as the 'basic rest activity cycle'. This cycle is called the Ultradian Rhythm and is controlled by our human biological clock.

By respecting and paying heed to this natural rhythm, you will be more efficient and creative in what you do.

Your stress levels will gradually decrease and this will have a powerful positive effect on your physical and mental health.

The **activity part** of the cycle lasts about 90–120 minutes. During this time, we are alert, able to focus and concentrate, on the ball and performing at our best.

Usually, after that period of time, our energy begins to wane and we are less clear-headed or focused – we lose a bit of our momentum, concentration and motivation. We may even feel drowsy. As you would expect, our performance drops.

This is our body's way of telling us that we are entering the **rest part** of the cycle (of the Ultradian Rhythm). This part of the cycle lasts about 7–10 minutes and we need to take time out to switch off our active, busy brain. During this time, our body needs to relax, replenish its energy and alertness, rejuvenate, and rebalance itself.

You can disturb your body's natural rhythm

Our basic rest activity cycle (BRAC) can become disturbed when we push our body to keep going despite it signalling to us that it needs a rest.

You may reach for the coffee to give you false energy. Doing this too often is like hitting the overworked and exhausted donkey with a stick to make him run faster, rather than giving him a break. This will eventually make you feel more distressed, harassed, and stressed.

You can get locked into overdrive

If we continue in an overdrive pattern for days, weeks, months and maybe years, we get locked into that pattern and it becomes our way of life. After some time, our body stops functioning properly – maybe we can't sleep so easily and can't stop worrying. Even when we have time for ourselves, we may feel restless, agitated and ill at ease.

When we are out of balance in this way, we may look outside, rather than inside, ourselves for reasons. If this state of affairs continues, it will lead to exhaustion, and, ultimately, it will damage our health.

Feel renewed – follow your ultradian rhythm

If you work according to your natural rhythm, you need to take a short rest period of 7–10 minutes every hour or two.

Be good to yourself

No one will look after you like you!

The next time your body signals to you that it is entering the **rest phase**, go with it and take a break instead of driving yourself to keep going. Afterwards, you will feel rejuvenated and more on the ball.

You will perform better and find it easier to learn and be more creative. You will also have more clarity when making important decisions.

Metaphorical story – The Overworked Donkey

No one will thank you for killing yourself.

It will be helpful to sit down and relax and read this metaphorical story about the Overworked Donkey – it has many truths to give you.

A man called Mr Rumbleton owned a small farm and lived off the land.

He decided to build a bigger storage shed for his winter harvest and use stones from the river bed for his building. The river bed was a good mile-and-a-half from his house. He bought a beautiful good-natured donkey and a cart to carry the stones up from the river.

The donkey was a lovely light brown colour with distinguishing white marks on his face. This donkey was healthy, strong and full of energy, playfulness and trust.

Mr Rumbleton worked the donkey from morning until noon each day carrying the stones. From noon until nightfall he hired the donkey out to Mr Egglebottom to work in his fields, ploughing the hard earth.

Day by day, from dawn to noon, the donkey carried heavy loads of stones from the river bed to Mr. Rumbleton's home without a break.

From noon to dusk, the donkey dragged the heavy plough through Mr Egglebottom's fields, turning over the hard dry earth. Ploughing fields was a job for a strong horse and not a donkey.

When the heavy load of stones the donkey pulled from the river slowed him, Mr Rumbleton kicked and beat him until he bled.

Each night, the donkey was locked in a pen with barely enough food and water to sustain him. He grew weaker and weaker every day. Every step became an effort to him. His once-shiny coat became sparse and mangy. His hooves were lacerated, and painful to walk on. He developed sores all over his body. He stumbled as he walked and fell sometimes, pulling the heavy cart.

He held his head low under his burden. He no longer sniffed the breeze or the sweet meadow smells or looked at the beautiful skies. The sun and moon and stars were a distant memory to him, leaving him feeling bereft and lost.

One night as he lay forlorn in the pen, hardly able to move, he felt compelled to drag himself up and walk to the pen gate. With great effort in the dark of night, he managed to yank the gate open with his mouth and steal out.

He grabbed some soft dew-drenched grass to eat as he struggled forward across the fields. He knew he had to keep going in order to escape.

All night long, exerting himself to the utmost, he struggled across fields and ditches.

He had to knock down a gate and two fences to follow his chosen direction. He knew instinctively which direction he wanted to take despite it being all new territory to him.

When dawn broke, he was standing close to Mary Dell's stone cottage. Mary Dell ran a small farm and sanctuary for mistreated and distressed animals. She welcomed the donkey gladly and so did her seven energetic, friendly children.

In no time at all, the donkey grew stronger and healthier. He helped out gladly on the farm with the other animals. He had time to play in the lush green fields with his friends. He had lots of time to sniff and eat his dewy grass, clover and daisies. He had lots of time to stand still and dream donkey dreams. He started to make his lovely braying sounds again. He was happy.

When Mr Rumbleton and Mr Egglebottom discovered that the donkey had escaped, they were enraged. They searched in vain for him. Eventually, they had to give up the search. They both agreed that he was a useless donkey, anyway, and no great loss.

Make the best use your rest cycle

There are many ways to get the most out of these 7–10 minute rest periods. It's important that you completely disengage from the work you have been doing – neither thinking about it nor talking about it. Take a few quiet moments for yourself where you can be comfortable. Perhaps do some relaxing breathing (see page 10) or even have a nice cup of tea.

Try any of the following exercises, alternating them if and when you please. Any of them will replenish, relax and rejuvenate you. You will be able to concentrate much better afterwards.

Like anything worthwhile, the more you practise them, the more quickly they will become part of your daily life, bringing you untold benefits.

Exercise 1   Create a fantasy energising place for yourself

You can instantly visit your fantasy place during your mini-breaks.

Close your eyes. Take a few relaxing breaths first. Release any tension from your body.

Now create a place that brings comfort to you and makes you happy.

As you become more involved in your picture, your body will relax more and more.

1 Picture yourself in the midst of the most *relaxing* beautiful surroundings. It can be an imaginary place or a real one where you went on holiday or which you have visited. It might be somewhere that you would like to visit, such as a beautiful seashore, a tropical island, a majestic waterfall, a golden desert, or a special mountain top.

2 As you picture this scene, imagine that you are there now – right now – living this experience, involving your senses and sensations to the full.

3 **What exactly do you see there?** Clear blue skies – sunlight dancing on the earth around you – breathtaking scenery – golden sands – sparkling blue sea?

4 **What can you hear in your beautiful landscape?** Beautiful music – the sound of the sea – the gentle song of birds – the whisper of the wind – the sound of a waterfall?

5 **What can you smell in your beautiful landscape?** Beautiful scent from the flowers – the smell of the sea air?

6 **What can you feel?** The warm sun on your skin – the gentle summer breeze on your face – the springy grass beneath your bare feet – the warm waters of the sea or rock pool on your skin?

7 **What does it feel like to be there?** What kind of feelings does this scene evoke in you? Calmness – peace – a feeling of joy or comfort? Feel those special feelings as if you were there now – *enjoy those feelings, savour them, live them for a little while.*

The more you do this exercise, the more quickly and profoundly deep you will feel those good, relaxing, energising feelings.

Exercise 2   Listen to light music

You might listen to some light gentle music and have a peaceful, happy daydream for yourself — no heavy metal!

Exercise 3   Meditation exercises

There are many very simple meditation exercises that will bring you peace and rejuvenate you.

See Resource 5 on Meditation Exercises in *Part Two*.
Pick one – give it a try – or feel free to create your own.

Important reminder No. 1
Listen to the wisdom of your body – take a mini-break at least 2–3 times a day for 7–10 minutes.

9
The Good Fruit Of Changing Unhelpful Views

Your views and your expectations – are they realistic?

We can have distorted views of situations and we can have unrealistic expectations of ourselves and others.

Both of these can trap us in stress.

Therefore, it is really important that you gain a wider understanding and awareness of the part your *perspective* and *expectations* play in your stress levels.

An illustrative scenario

James and Lisa

When James and Lisa got married two years ago, everyone said that it was 'a match made in heaven'. Lisa's parents are conventional and very religious, believing that marriage is for life. Lisa is getting scared of James – he is bullying, controlling and intensely jealous of her. At home, he constantly puts her down and has unwarranted rages. In public, James is a gentleman. Lisa is very unhappy and realises that she has made a grave mistake. She wants to get out of the marriage.

Lisa's view and expectations

- **Lisa's view** – Lisa thinks that her parents will disown her and that they will be very disappointed with her if she leaves James as they think James is marvellous.

- **Lisa's expectations** – She expects herself to honour the sanctity of marriage and be a dutiful wife to James despite his frightening behaviour. Lisa also expects herself to be a dutiful daughter and fulfil her parents' beliefs and expectations.
- **More of Lisa's views** – If she leaves James, it will bring shame on the family and it will be all her fault. She has come to the conclusion that people are going to think badly of her if she leaves the marriage and that she will have no friends.

She is extremely stressed, anxious and fearful, and feels trapped. She is losing her confidence and self-esteem.

She feels she has no one to turn to.

The good fruit of Lisa adopting a more balanced view and more realistic expectations

- **Lisa's new realistic expectations** – She can realise that it is her basic human right to be in a non-abusive relationship and to expect respect, happiness and fulfilment from that relationship.

  She can also realise that her parents' expectations belong to them and not to her and it is her life and hers to live.

  She can also realise that being able to leave her abusive relationship is a realistic expectation and is the best and most honest thing she can do for herself.

- **Lisa's new balanced views** – She can adopt a point of view that being able to admit her mistake in marrying James is brave and nothing to be ashamed of.

  She can reaffirm to herself that her parents love her even if they don't approve of her leaving the marriage.

  She can use the opportunity to talk honestly about her and James's relationship to her parents, close family and a best friend, which will help her. It will give her parents a more honest perspective.

  Even if her parents are disappointed, she can take the view that their reaction is not her problem. She is not her parents.

From a fresh viewpoint, Lisa can see that, if her friends are real friends, they will remain her friends. If not, she will survive, cope and even get stronger and find other friends.

She can take the view that, even if it is a stressful and sad time, she will still be okay and much wiser and happier, and she can seek professional help if she needs it.

Once Lisa has these new perspectives and realistic expectations, she will be less fearful and, feeling more supported and more confident in herself, she will have the strength to take the right action.

If you can change how you look at a situation, put a more positive slant on it and alter your unrealistic expectations of yourself and of others, you can change how you feel about it and you will feel more empowered.

Also, you will be inclined to find a better way to deal with the situation.

This will give you more confidence and you will feel more in control.

The truth or unrealistic thinking – which is it?

Although your view of many stressful situations may be based on truth and reality, unfortunately most of us harbour some repetitive distorted ways of thinking that create a lot of stress for us and for others too. These unhelpful thinking patterns are described as *Cognitive Distortions* because they distort our view of reality. They trap us in stress and self-sabotaging behaviour and often in unrealistic expectations.

Many thought patterns we developed as children and as young adults are great and helpful. However, many are more than a bit off-kilter and cause us to view things in repetitive, rigid and unhelpful ways. This can leave us feeling trapped, guilty, angry, frustrated, upset or hard-done-by.

The fallout from our Cognitive Distortions

Our *Cognitive Distortions* have a major negative impact on how we *interpret* our experiences.

These patterns appear so normal to us that we rarely think of them as being skewed and so we rarely challenge them.

They usually trigger negative emotional reactions in us to specific situations, people and experiences. The more repetitive and rigid these patterns are, the more they distort our views of reality.

The power of even one change

When you change even just one of your *Cognitive Distortions*, it will release a bundle of stress from your life.

You will be able to take a more optimistic view of certain situations.

You will be able to deal with these situations in a more resourceful way.

Particular *Cognitive Distortions* make us view things in specific ways

For example, if you have a pattern of over-generalising/jumping to the wrong conclusion, you can have one bad experience with someone and come to the crazy conclusion that every future experience with them is going to be bad or worse.

As for your expectations of yourself, don't always expect to be perfect! That is unrealistic.

It is also unrealistic always to expect others to be perfect.

In *Part Two* of this book, in Resources 1, 2 and 3, you will find information on the most common *Cognitive Distortions* that plague many us.

These Resources will enable you to:

a Identify any of your own unhelpful cognitive distortions.

b Change these distortive patterns.

c Adopt more balanced views.

d Do a bit of Cognitive Behavioural Therapy (CBT) on yourself when you need it, using our quick and simple format.

Important reminder No. 1
Look closely at your views and expectations in situations that you react strongly to.

Important reminder No. 2
Remember that it takes courage to move out from familiar to unfamiliar territory. You will find yourself coming up with all sorts of reasons why a new point of view and way of dealing with the situation/person won't work. **Take note** – we shall always try to justify our way of thinking in order to defend our own, albeit unhelpful, conditioned response – don't fall into that trap!

Important reminder No. 3
To enable you to change your perspective or unrealistic expectation, it often helps to put yourself in another's shoes – to give yourself a different perspective. This can increase understanding and empathy for others and for yourself.

Important final reminder
Whenever you want to change your perspective, remember that you need to be in a calm state of mind.

10
Talk Kindly To Yourself – Feel Less Stressed

Talk kindly to yourself like a true friend

Our inner voice or 'self talk' refers to what we say to ourselves about ourselves in our mind or even out loud. Our self talk is also about what we say to ourselves about others in our mind. Our self talk can be positive or negative, loving or critical and full of put-downs, such as, 'I'm stupid, an idiot, fat, ugly.'

The amazing power of our self talk

> Our self talk can empower or diminish us because our whole way of being, feeling and behaving is influenced by how we talk to ourselves.

Sometimes we beat ourselves up more than we encourage ourselves or talk kindly to ourselves. The repercussions of doing this to ourselves take an enormous toll on our confidence and self-esteem and raise accordingly our stress level.

Sometimes, in our head, we can also put others down unfairly by repeated unjust and harsh criticism.

Our unconscious mind absorbs our repetitive self talk

What we habitually tell ourselves and really believe to be true is taken as truth in our subconscious mind because it cannot differentiate truth from falsehood. This will just create and reinforce more negative beliefs about ourselves.

We need to be our own best friend and start talking very kindly to ourselves. Remember, all human beings are unique, are equally valuable and deserving of fair treatment, equality and respect. You are just as special and precious as anyone else, irrespective of what you think you can and can't do or what you have or have not done.

We can all reclaim our power and confidence and this is a good place to start – talking kindly to ourselves.

Optimistic self talk can lift our spirits

Our optimistic, helpful self talk can empower us, no matter what has happened, and it helps if we can be our own true friend.

Optimistic self talk can lift your spirits and bring health-promoting hormones into your blood.

Our encouraging self talk creates a more optimistic state of mind and emotions and enables us to function better. We all know how good it feels if someone is there for us when things go wrong – someone who will stand by us and be our true friend. You can now do that for yourself and always be there for yourself.

Your positive self talk can give you hope, increase your confidence and creativity and help you to do your best in situations. It promotes optimism and emotional development and helps you get more out of life and your relationships.

Our negative self talk can diminish us

When we become our own harsh judge, rather than our own best friend, our self-esteem and confidence will suffer.

If we continually tell ourselves untruths, the more stressed out we shall be. It can sabotage you on every level; sap your confidence; and erode your self-esteem.

Negative self talk can block your creativity, stop you from seeing things clearly and prevent you from solving your problems. It can de-motivate and exhaust you and make you feel defeated and hopeless, as well as lowering your immune system.

Negative self talk often arises spontaneously and can become a bad habit. It is more likely to occur when you are feeling anxious or upset, as you saw in Mark's case (chapter five).

> Repetitive negative self talk will flood your body with stress hormones and play havoc with your health, happiness and relationships.
>
> The Repetitive Messages of negative self talk can create a pessimistic state of mind and leave you feeling anxious, even deflated and depressed.
>
> It can blind you to the good you already have in your life.

Repetitive negative self talk, including criticism, harsh judgment and put-downs, is fuelled by misguided and untrue beliefs most likely adopted in childhood. **They do not reflect who you really are. Don't give away your confidence and power to them!**

Begin to recognise your negative self talk

Don't be discouraged if you have a lot of negative self talk – know that it is a very common human trait. You can begin to change it now and you will get immediate positive results.

Exercise I

1 Pick one specific recurring situation that causes you stress (write it down for clarity if you wish).

2 What is your self talk in this situation, i.e. what exactly are you telling yourself? Is your self talk critical? Is it full of harsh judgment, put-downs, self-blame and self-condemnation? Is your self talk about others the same?

3 Is your negative self talk making you feel bad, demoralised, hopeless, distressed, depressed, more stressed out?

Loosen the grip of this negative self talk

Exercise 2

1 If you find yourself putting yourself down because you haven't lived up to your own or others expectations – STOP. Realise we can all make mistakes and we need to acknowledge them and we can learn whatever lesson we need to.
2 Breathe; release those negative thoughts like black polluted smoke from your mind and body with your relaxing out breath.
3 Now talk optimistically to yourself in a loving supportive way as you would do to a very dear best friend.

Gain control over your negative self talk

Whenever you hear yourself putting yourself down, do the following powerful exercise. The more you do this exercise, the more quickly you will eliminate this unhelpful pattern.

Exercise 3

First of all, relax yourself by taking some relaxing breaths.

- Imagine your self-talk taking the form of an ugly little imp dressed in black with a long snout, bulgy eyes, a big mouth with no teeth and smelly breath!
- Imagine him with a squeaky, high-pitched, irritating voice yapping at your heels, trying to put you down and make you feel bad about yourself (how annoyed and cross would you feel!).
- Now, in your head, shout at him to get out of your sight and not come back. A little kick up the backside would send him on his way!
- Watch and hear him scuttle off, looking behind him to make sure you are not following him with the toe of your shoe!
  OR
- Shrink him down in your imagination to be a small wriggly worm that a big black crow comes and eats up.

Important reminder No. 1

Try to get into the habit of confronting your repetitive negative self talk and recognising it for what it is – an old faulty programme in your brain.

Important reminder No. 2

Changing your negative self talk is a must if you want to have a happier life.

Final reminder

Positive self talk creates a more positive state of mind and positive emotions. It helps you do your best in any situation.

11
Make Gratitude And Generosity Your Gifts

Make gratitude your gift to yourself

A spirit of gratitude and generosity will not only reduce your worries, it will open your heart and help you cultivate a happier and more optimistic life for yourself.

Gratitude brings happy hormones (endorphins) into our blood, creating the 'feel good factor' and helping us build a healthy immune system.

Gratitude makes you happy and optimistic

When worried, we often tend to focus only on what is going wrong for us or on what we lack.

Gratitude is heartfelt appreciation for all we already have. The more often you show gratitude, the more positively you begin to think and negative thought patterns weaken and begin to melt away.

Gratitude lessens our feelings of insecurity and makes us happier. A spirit of gratitude builds our confidence and feeling of self-worth.

It makes us more compassionate and ready to appreciate ourselves and others more.

You already have many gifts in life

There is so much in your everyday life that you can be grateful for. It is an on-the-spot gift you can give yourself and others anytime, anywhere.

When you wake each morning, you could show gratitude for a new day. This will put you in a positive frame of mind. We can be grateful for the air we breathe, the sun that shines for us, every flower and tree that grows for us, the wind that blows, the beauty of the earth all around us, the rain that makes our land alive and gives us water.

You can be grateful if you can walk, talk, see and hear; grateful because you have somewhere to live, food to eat, and clothes to wear; grateful that others care about you – family, a friend, your cat or dog.

The list is never ending. The more things you appreciate in your life, the more likely you are to find reasons to be thankful.

Be grateful for beautiful you!

No matter what kind of day you have had, you can always find something to be grateful for. This will lift your spirits a little and make you smile.

Don't forget to give gratitude to yourself many times in your day – gratitude for all your beautiful qualities and capabilities; gratitude for the times you try when you don't feel like it; the things you do when you don't feel up to it; the kind things you do for yourself and others; for the painful lessons you have learned – and maybe for cooking the best cake ever!

Showing gratitude to others lifts their spirits

We can show gratitude to others by letting them know when we are grateful.

We can feel gratitude towards others, for the mere fact of their existence or because they give us a smile, or a helping hand.

Showing gratitude to others gives us a sense of peace and connection with them. Giving a smile, a word of kindness, a helping hand, or a bit of cheer to others can brighten up their day.

Gratitude and appreciation need to be freely given without expectation of getting anything in return. However, you are always rewarded because giving gratitude always makes you feel better.

> Give gratitude as many times as you can and you will be amazed at the many positive changes that take place in your life.
>
> Gratitude needs to be practised on a day-to-day basis in order to grow.

Gratitude helps our generosity to grow

The spirit of generosity is about being big-hearted, good-hearted, warm-hearted, magnanimous.

Generosity comes from the heart. When you open your heart to others in a spirit of generosity, you truly give of yourself (it doesn't mean allowing ourselves to be taken advantage of). A generous heart does not give out of guilt or to win acclaim, recognition or fame – generosity comes from love; the love that wants to reach out to ourselves and others.

> Developing a generous spirit will make you happier and more positive and you will appreciate yourself and others more.
>
> Developing a spirit of generosity will make you kinder and more understanding of yourself and others.
>
> The hearts of others will open to you too – you will get more happiness out of life.
>
> If you are generous to yourself and to others, you will be amazed at how much better you feel.
>
> Love will blossom in your life.

First be generous to yourself

First of all, you need to be generous to yourself.

That means taking care of your health – mentally, emotionally and spiritually. Be generous to yourself when you make mistakes or don't live up to your own expectations. Be generous to yourself when things go wrong in your life. Be generous and give yourself time for laughter and fun and doing something you enjoy. Be generous to yourself for being who you are – a unique, beautiful spark of life. Be generous to yourself by opening your heart to honesty and helping yourself learn life's lessons.

Be generous to others

Many of us associate generosity with giving money and indeed it can be about sharing our good fortune with others who are not as fortunate.

Generosity can also be about giving someone the benefit of the doubt – a second chance – and trying to understand another's predicament. It can be about sharing and giving a helping hand to others.

It can be about giving a bit of tolerance, your time, affection, attention, a listening ear, a truthful opinion when asked, kindness or support to another who needs it.

Generosity is about letting go of grudges, petty differences and harsh judgments of others. It's about being emotionally generous, sharing power, knowledge and credit with others.

It is about being able to forgive yourself and others. It can be about giving a bit of cheer and goodwill, even a smile, a hug, the time of day to others.

Generosity can be about standing up for others, too, when needs be and being able to put ourselves on the line rather than sitting on the fence.

A spirit of generosity helps us to become less self-absorbed, and more at peace with ourselves and others.

To develop a spirit of generosity, you need to practise it on a daily basis as many times as you can.

In this way, your spirit of generosity and big-heartedness will grow.

An exercise to increase feelings of appreciation and happiness

Do this exercise often and your feelings of happiness and optimism will grow bigger and bigger!

Take a few relaxing breaths first.

- Bring to mind now something that you are truly grateful for and really appreciate. It might be a friend, a family member or someone who loves you; it might be gratitude for something you have in your life – a house, a garden, a car, a job you like.

- Put your hand over your heart and focus on your heart for a moment, giving thanks.

- Close your eyes and dwell on this person/gift for a few moments, using all your senses and feelings. Now notice the warm sensations – the 'feel good factor' – you get when you bring this to mind. Be aware of how these happy sensations make you feel. Notice that you begin to smile. Notice how your body begins to let go and relax. Give thanks again for this person/gift that brings joy into your life.

Important reminder No. 1
Cultivate a spirit of gratitude by giving appreciation daily for some of the good things you have in your life.

Important reminder No. 2
Gratitude opens our heart and brings happy hormones (endorphins) into our blood, creating the 'feel good factor' and making you feel better about yourself.

Important reminder No. 3
Be big-hearted, warm and generous – you will reap many benefits.

12
Face Your Worries

Don't drag your worries along with you

We have to know how and when to let go of our worries. When we worry about the same thing over and over again, it often means that we are avoiding taking proper action or we are refusing to accept what we can't change.

Wake up to the things and people that stress you

You need to identify the situations and people that stress you in your life.

This means being aware of your thoughts, feelings and reactions to them.

This will allow you to choose the best way to deal with the situations and people involved.

Don't suffer alone with major stressors

Seeking professional help when you need it is about reasserting power over your own life. Many of our ongoing problems such as relationship difficulties, or being bullied, can leave us sad and disillusioned, as well as stressed. These, if unresolved, can keep us in a state of high stress, anxiety, anger and sadness. Time is too precious to get stuck in that – the problems need resolving.

Why problems in our life need resolving

Our unresolved problems can drain us emotionally and physically. They trap us, and prevent us from moving forward in our lives.

Hiding from our problems is not an option; it creates even more stress and unhappiness. It doesn't matter how much we hide from or ignore our problems – they will always find us, sit beside us and persecute us until we resolve them somehow!

Let's face it, more often than not we see our problems as bigger than they really are or just unique to us. This stops us from facing them and resolving them or getting help with them.

Our unresolved problems will not go away; they will continue to cause worry and unhappiness in our life.

When we resolve them or come to terms with them, a great weight is lifted off our shoulders.

The next chapter will show you how you can identify and resolve your problems and dilemmas.

13
Identify And Resolve Your Problems And Dilemmas

Identify your problems

Some of our problems are complex and have many aspects to them, yet with good problem-solving skills we can resolve them. Many, however, are very simple, yet none the less, if unresolved, they can cause a lot of stress.

A quick guide to help you identify your stressors

Sit down where you won't be disturbed for 10–15 minutes.
Have a pen and paper to hand.
Do relaxing breathing to calm yourself.

1 Off the top of your head, quickly list all the situations, things or people that make you anxious, worried, upset, annoyed or angry at the moment. Don't dwell on anything – just write your list quickly.

2 Divide the list into two sections. The most bothersome situations and the least bothersome ones.

Look at your *least* bothersome list first.

Gradually begin to eliminate some of these minor stressors – you will be surprised at how much better you begin to feel.

Many minor stressors can be quick and simple to resolve, perhaps by being more organised, managing your time and resources better, or eliminating unnecessary hassles from your life.

If you can, resolve some of your minor stressors and sort out your priorities. This will put you in a better frame of mind to tackle a major stressor.

How you view your problem is important

1 Focus on the solution to your problem or dilemma, not on the problem

Whenever you're faced with a problem or difficulty, accept responsibility for it – you are the one who has it. Focus on finding a good solution. This relieves some stress, empowers you and changes your perspective.

If you focus too much on the problem, you will increase your stress levels and you may fail to see opportunities and solutions.

2 Create a positive attitude and positive expectation

When we are in a good mood or 'loved up', we cope more easily with everyday challenges. When we are in a negative mood, even small challenges can seem too much.

Our moods or state of mind greatly influence how we perceive and interpret situations and that is why they can either limit or empower us. It is good to bear this in mind when we are looking for resolutions to our problems or making positive changes.

Focusing your energy on finding a solution engages your creative, imaginative brain as well as your sophisticated, rational brain.

It increases your confidence and 'feel good factor'.

Now make yourself comfortable, relax and enjoy reading this metaphorical problem-solving story. Let it empower you and put a smile on your face!

The Old Captured Bear

A great brown grizzly bear was captured and put to live in a park, which seemed to have everything the bear needed and wanted – food, shelter and a space to roam in. The park was enclosed by a very strong reinforced concrete wall with a foot of barbed-wire on top of the wall to prevent the bear from escaping.

The bear soon became distraught, angry and frustrated because he hated being in the park. He wanted the freedom of the forests, the rivers and the mountains – his real home. He roared and cried out and moaned in his sleep every night, so distressed was he.

A small black rat that lived in the park heard him roar and cry out every night. The rat got curious and mustered up the courage to talk to the bear.

'Why are you roaring and crying and moaning every night in your sleep?' asked the rat.

The bear felt like swiping the rat with his great paw but desperation drove him to tell the rat of his frustration and entrapment.

'I can show you a way out,' said the rat, 'but once I show you there is no room for dithering.'

That night, the rat arrived with a small army of sharp-toothed brown rat friends. They gnawed away a large section from the vicious barbed-wire fence.

'Now get your big bear's hairy arse up on the wall and over the fence quickly!' shouted the black rat. 'It's your chance now – no dithering.'

The bear made a thundering dash for it, grunting and puffing. He let out a yelp as the vicious barbed-wire dug into his flesh, yet he held on fast with his big body swaying and quivering in mid-air.

'You sure are a great sight, bear,' shouted the black rat. 'Keep going – keep going – no dithering.'

With a lot of struggling and blustering and grunting, the bear somehow managed to scramble through the hole made in the barbed-wire fence at the top of the wall and threw himself onto the ground below with a great thud.

The rats gasped, covered their eyes with their little paws and squealed.

The bear got up, shook himself, and raced towards the forest and hills as fast as he could. You could hear his loud roars of delight as he charged along. You could hear the black rat's squeals of delight as he saw the bear run to freedom.

Tips for resolving bigger problems

Pick one specific problem to work on at a time.

Set aside a special time for yourself to look at your problem.

Take a few relaxing breaths to bring yourself to a place of calmness.

Step 1 Identify the problem

Example – Worried about being made redundant

- Identify the problem, define it clearly, describe it clearly and write it down.
- Look at every aspect of your problem – the good parts and the bad.
- Now write down exactly what you are worrying about, for example: 'I am worrying because I was made redundant and I can't find a job.'
- Ask yourself 'What is it about this that is a worry to me?' You may answer that you won't have enough money to live on or pay your bills; that you will be bored and have nothing to do; that you will be lonely and isolated; that you will never find a job again; that people might judge you harshly.
- Describe how each aspect of your problem is affecting your life and what will happen if you allow the problem to continue.

Step 2 Find a resolution

Begin by brainstorming and, if necessary, break the problem into small, practical, manageable steps.

Identify several possible solutions and evaluate each solution – the pros and cons of each one.

- Choose your best solution. Look at it carefully and see exactly what you will gain from that solution and also what you might lose.
- Write your solution down very clearly. Define what you want to happen or achieve.
- Develop a good, time-specific plan of action to be taken in measurable steps that will help you to reach a resolution and take action as soon as possible.

Break problems down into their different aspects and find solutions for each aspect.

When we face our problems and break them down into time-specific, manageable steps, we can resolve them much more easily than we imagined.

Break your problem down into its different aspects.

Then break each aspect down into time-specific, manageable, measurable steps.

Apply problem-solving techniques to each aspect.

This will enable you to find the best solution to the overall problem.

When it comes to resolving your problems – take some action straight away.

Procrastination drinks your confidence and eats away good opportunities.

The following diagram illustrates how to do this.

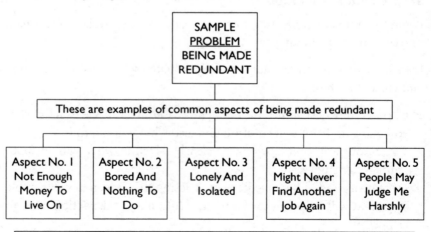

SAMPLE
PROBLEM
BEING MADE
REDUNDANT

These are examples of common aspects of being made redundant

Aspect No. 1	Aspect No. 2	Aspect No. 3	Aspect No. 4	Aspect No. 5
Not Enough Money To Live On	Bored And Nothing To Do	Lonely And Isolated	Might Never Find Another Job Again	People May Judge Me Harshly

Set a specific, realistic time to take the necessary steps required for each Aspect.

Take action on each Aspect as soon as is possible.

Aspect no. 1 – Not enough money to live on
- Assess your financial incomings and outgoings
- Calculate the deficit
- Look at any opportunities to make extra cash
- Seek professional financial advice

Aspect no. 2 – Bored and nothing to do
- Consider doing some things or jobs that you have put off
- Consider learning a new skill, like cooking or gardening
- Consider voluntary work
- Investigate what is going on in your community

Aspect No. 3 – Lonely and isolated
- Join a group in your community and make new friends
- Catch up with family or old friends
- Get out, go for a walk in the park or countryside every day
- Take up a hobby

Aspect No. 4 – Might never find another job again
- Brush up on your CV and job application writing skills – get help if needed
- Brush up your networking skills
- Seek out confidence-building and assertiveness skills
- Seek free computer training courses in the community
- Seek free career advice and consider alternative career option
- Seek help with interview techniques

Aspect No. 5 – People may judge me harshly
- Recognise that most people generally don't have this attitude
- Recognise that it is not your fault, it's happening to many people
- Our book contains many resources to relieve your stress and build your confidence and self-esteem
- If people do judge you harshly, it is their negative pattern and NOT yours!

Let go of past worries

Sometimes a situation from the past that **we cannot do anything about** may continue to worry us and even make us feel guilty.

The following exercise will help you reduce your **anxiety** and perhaps give you more clarity regarding any such situations, thus enabling you to *come to terms* with them or *resolve* them where possible.

Find a comfortable place to sit or lie down where you won't be disturbed. Do a relaxing breathing exercise for a few moments.

The Old Black Heavy Smelly Coat

Let an old black, heavy, smelly coat represent whichever past stressful situation that is still worrying you and you can do nothing about.

- Imagine walking along a path through a field in the early morning.
- The sky overhead is a dull grey without even one ray of sunshine peeping through.
- The grass feels rough and dry against your bare feet as you walk along.
- You listen in vain for the song of a bird but all you hear is the persistent cawing of crows coming from the trees at the side of the field.
- The air feels heavy and sultry and there is not even a hint of a breeze. You feel droplets of sweat trickling down your face and back.
- You feel exhausted, overwhelmed and hot.
- You are wearing an old heavy black coat that is dragging you down. It smells stale and fusty.

- As you approach the end of the path, you notice a bonfire burning brightly on your right.

- You walk over to look at it and you are mesmerised by its leaping orange, red and blue flames and the sound of it crackling and spitting.
- Despite being hot and sweaty, you find the heat and the energy of the burning fire comforting and reassuring.
- Deliberately and with determination, you take off your old black, heavy, smelly coat and throw it into the leaping flames of the burning fire. You watch as the flames seize and engulf your old black, heavy, smelly coat and rapidly reduce it to ashes.
- A wave of relief sweeps over you and you walk light-heartedly towards a golden bridge that is close by your path.

- You stand awhile on the golden bridge, looking into the clear fast-flowing river below, and then walk across it into a beautiful sunlit meadow.

Now close your eyes and take a few relaxing breaths.

As you breathe in, imagine breathing the pure light of love into your heart for a few moments.

Thank your beautiful heart for being there for you 24 hours of every day of your life.

Important reminder No. 1
Face your problems or you will have to drag them along with you.

14
Know Your Priorities – Become Self-Aware

The great importance of self-awareness

Self-awareness is about knowing who and what are really important to you in life. This will prevent you putting too much of your energy and time into things or people that matter little in your life. So many times we look back on aspects of our lives and wish we had given more time and commitment to more important things or people in our lives.

Self-awareness is about knowing what your own beliefs and expectations are. It is about knowing your priorities in life, what makes you happy in life or what makes you excited and gives you joy and fulfilment. It is about having a clear insight into your strengths and talents, so that you can enhance your talents and strengthen your weaknesses.

If you feel as though your life is slipping out of control, or that you have missed the right turn, or taken a wrong turn, or have no clear focus and feel dissatisfied, identifying your real priorities is the first step in the right direction.

Taking action to achieve your priorities is the second and final step.

Whatever your important priorities are, remember that taking good care of your mental, emotional, physical and spiritual health is an absolute must for you to be happy.

Turn not away from your heartfelt desires

The human spirit is a joyful one and you deserve to be happy and follow your dreams. Be honest with yourself, recognise your wants and needs, and listen to your own heartfelt feelings and desires. If you give time and commitment and take positive action to fulfil them, you take a step towards creating a happier and more meaningful life for yourself.

The ability to prioritise and reach for what is important to you in life is vital to your health and well-being. Everyone feels better when they are doing what they are happy with and what is important to them, be that a particular job, children, relationship, marriage, hobbies or travel.

> We need to separate what is important from what is irrelevant or simply a distraction in our life.

Each of us is an individual and each one of us will have our own priorities – and that is fine. Some of our priorities may change over the years while some remain the same. Some of our priorities are big but we also have small ones – and we need to pay heed to them, too.

Examples of common priorities people have

A loving relationship, friendships, family, children

Having a nice home and a nice area to live in

Financial security

Education, a career, a particular type of job

Developing abilities and talents

Helping the community, the environment, nature

A good social life, having fun, hobbies, travel

Self-development

Sometimes we don't know our priorities!

The following little exercise might help to identify your priorities.

Sit down and relax – your mind will be more creative and focused when you are relaxed.

List your priorities and rate each on a scale of 1–10, with 10 being the most important. Each will hold a different value for you.

- Ask yourself 'What is the single most important heartfelt desire in my life?
- What would really make me happy?'
- How would you rate this priority on a scale of 1–10?
- Imagine now that you already have this: how would it make you feel – happy/confident/proud/excited/secure?
- Ask yourself 'What would this heartfelt desire give me?' For example would you have more money/recognition/freedom/choices?
- Ask yourself 'Are there any disadvantages in fulfilling this heartfelt desire?' For example would you have too much responsibility/too little time for family or important relationships?
- How would you rate this heartfelt desire now – is it higher or lower than your original rating?

You can do this with all the priorities on your list.

Once you have found out your single most important priority in life, determine your next most important one. Find two or three areas of your life that you need to examine to ensure your happiness.

A metaphorical story to highlight the importance of your priorities

Sit down, relax and put your feet up. Now slowly read this metaphorical story.

The Blackbirds

It was spring and the earth began to dance with new life and throw out new shoots, fresh green leaves and fragrant, delicate blossoms.

A pair of blackbirds began to build their nest in a fresh leafy tree in a park. A pair of jays, a pair of thrushes, and a pair of woodpeckers were building their nests close by. There was plenty of soft moss, feathers and lamb's wool around for all the birds to line their nests with.

When the blackbirds had partially built their own nest, they left it unfinished and they began to help the jays, woodpeckers and thrushes to build their nests. The jays, woodpeckers and thrushes were perplexed as to why the blackbirds didn't seem to want to finish their own nest. Of course, they were delighted with such unexpected help. It gave them more time to play around and have a good time, knowing that the blackbirds were making their nests snug, secure and warm for them.

Soon the nests of the jays, woodpeckers and thrushes were finished and snug as could be while the blackbirds' nest was left dangling unfinished between two branches. The mother blackbird had to lay her eggs in a hurry so the blackbirds had to make do with the unfinished nest for their beautiful blue speckled eggs.

The blackbirds' eggs were now exposed to the cold night winds and passing predators, like the two jays and a hawk that hovered nearby waiting for their chance. As a result, the blackbirds had to sit on their unfinished nest every second of the day and night to protect their eggs from being eaten.

By the time the eggs hatched out and four baby chicks emerged from the shells, the blackbirds were thin, dishevelled and exhausted. The new baby chicks' movements made the unfinished nest even more unstable and wobbly. The chicks became desperate for food and both exhausted blackbird parents flew into a nearby field, searching for food for themselves and their chicks.

With little warning, a great wind gathered force and blew fiercely among the trees. The blackbirds' badly made nest with the four baby chicks took to the air and landed in pieces on the ground below.

Bruised and frightened, the weak little blackbird chicks cried and wailed helplessly on the ground. They hid under some big leaves that were blown from the tree.

The parent blackbirds were broken-hearted to find their nest gone and their little baby chicks nowhere to be found. Their desperate cries and calls echoed around the trees. 'If only,' they said to each other, 'we had made a proper nest for our beautiful babes and fed them well, this would not have happened.' They were totally inconsolable.

The jays, woodpeckers and thrushes did not come to console the blackbirds or help them look for their little babies. It was by chance that the blackbirds heard their little chicks' mournful cries. They found them under the leaves, huddled together, trembling from fright and hunger.

The two resourceful blackbirds quickly found a safe hole in a big tall oak tree close by. They carried their little chicks to their new home in the oak tree. Very soon, the blackbirds had made the nest as snug as could be by lining it with dry moss and sheep's wool. They carried the choicest food to their beautiful chicks and ate plenty themselves. They all grew strong, happy and healthy and enjoyed a magical summer flight together.

Important reminder No. 1
Taking care of all aspects of your health is your first priority.

Important reminder No. 2
Honour your priorities by making the necessary arrangements to give time, energy and commitment to them.

15
Steps To
Achieve Your Goals

Set a goal and navigate your way to it

Setting yourself goals and achieving them are very important for your confidence, happiness and well-being, and great for enabling you to achieve your priorities, big and small.

Setting goals will help you to focus and direct your thoughts, time and energy into achieving your desires.

Properly set and clearly-defined goals, broken down into easy achievable steps, will motivate you to take action and turn your goals into reality.

Without goals, we drift off course, quickly lose our motivation, get disheartened, abandon ship and beat ourselves up. We try something else and repeat the same behaviour.

Tips for setting goals

When setting goals, it is important that your goals align with your values and beliefs.

For example, if you value truth and believe strongly in being a truthful person, you won't be happy having a job that leads you to trick and manipulate people!

- Make sure that your goals are important to you in your life.
- Goals need to be very clear and specific.

- Set goals for yourself that are realistic and achievable within a specific time-frame.

Write down a detailed description of your goals

- Write down what benefits your goals will give you – for example, money, security, happiness, contentment, better health, a sense of pride, doing something you love, interest, or enjoyment. This makes the goals clearer in your mind and easier to focus on and follow through.
- Break your goals down into achievable time-specific steps.
- You need to be able to measure your progress along the way.
  For example, if you want to find a job, one of your measurable steps towards it might be completing a good CV within 3 - 4 days.
- You need to devise a plan that will let you know when you have achieved your goals – so you can celebrate!

Visualise yourself as having already achieved your goals

Visualising your goals as if you have already achieved them is a great way to help bring them into reality and boost focus, motivation and determination.

Remember, our brain cannot tell the difference between something that's real and something imagined and will respond equally to both, giving you the drive you need.

Make your imagined goals as big, bright, bold and realistic as possible. See them – hear what people say – smell them – touch them!

Simple example of goal-setting

Mary lives alone. Mary has a full-time job and is home every day at 5 pm.

Mary has a goal to paint her *three-bedroom house* before she puts it on the market for sale in three months' time.

Mary feels that this will add value to the house, make it more desirable and sell more quickly. She feels that any prospective buyers will be drawn to her house when they see how nice it is. She needs to paint the house herself because of her financial situation.

Mary's plan for achieving her goal

Mary decides that her goal is to have her house painted by 20th May, which will be in two months' time. This, Mary feels, is a realistic and attainable goal.

Mary can now visualise herself as having achieved her goal and repeat her visualisation often!

How does Mary visualise her goal?

Mary makes herself comfortable and does some relaxing breathing for a few moments.

She imagines that all her rooms are now painted ...

She clearly imagines that the newly-painted rooms of her house look bright, cheerful and bring more light into the house and she herself feels lighter and happier as a result.

She imagines her house now having a nice, clean, fresh feel and smell to it.

She imagines lighting her special vanilla candle and enjoying sitting there for a few moments, admiring her beautiful newly-painted house. She feels real pride in her achievement and it's a great feeling. She congratulates herself on doing it so well and for being so organised about it.

She imagines her neighbour, Jean, coming in and being so surprised at how wonderful it looks and giving her a hug. In her mind's eye she can see herself getting many good offers for the house.

Action plan – taking achievable steps

Mary decides to paint **one room at a time**, starting with one of the spare bedrooms upstairs.

Mary estimates that she could paint that room in a day and decides that she will use this coming weekend (2 days) to paint her two spare bedrooms.

Mary then decides to use the following weekend to paint the bathroom and her own bedroom.

Mary decides to use the third weekend to paint her living room.

She realises she will be unable to paint her hall and stairway herself and needs to find someone who will paint on that Saturday of the 3rd weekend while she is painting the living room.

Mary plans to use the fourth weekend to paint her kitchen.

Steps Mary takes to reach her goal – planning ahead

- Mary decides to shop on her way from work tomorrow to get everything she needs to paint the two rooms.
- She makes a list that evening of what she needs to buy and chooses the colour of the paint.
- To save time cooking while painting, Mary plans to buy ready-made meals on Friday evening on her way home from work.
- Mary plans to start painting at 8 am on Saturday and 8 am on Sunday morning.
- To ensure that she will find someone to paint her hall on that third Saturday, Mary decides to pop over tonight and ask her neighbour for the telephone number of the painter who did such a marvellous job on her house.
- She rings him that evening and he agrees to paint the stairs and landing for her on that Saturday.

Mary takes action on all of the above and worked according to her plans

Mary acknowledges her step-by-step achievement

Mary finished in less than her allotted time. Mary felt good and proud of each achievement along the way. She admired each painted room and felt a real sense of joy and achievement. Now that it is complete, Mary is proud of her hard work and of how lovely her rooms look.

She strongly feels that when she puts her house on the market it will now have a better chance of being sold quickly. She gives herself a pat on the back and congratulates herself on achieving her goal and doing it so quickly and well.

Important reminder No. 1
Define your goals. Make sure that they are what you want and that they are attainable.

Important reminder No. 2
Give yourself a time-frame within which to achieve your goals.

Important reminder No. 3
Break your future goals into manageable projects. You can then break these projects down into smaller parts until you find some action that you can do **right now, however small the step.**

Important reminder No. 4
Visualise your goals as if you have already achieved them.

Important reminder No. 5
Acknowledge each achieved step along the way and feel good about it.

Important reminder No. 6
Reach your goal!

16
Let Your Heart Heal You

Your heart brain and your stress connection

Our heart is the seat of our emotions and deepest feelings. When we feel joy and love in our heart, it makes our world seem a happier place. When we feel sadness and despair, our heart sinks.

The reputable Institute of HeartMath has been carrying out advanced research for many years on our human heart. Their tried and tested findings give us the knowledge and tools to live a much less stressed, happier, healthier life.

HeartMath research concludes that:

- Our heart is not just a mere physical organ pumping blood but a 'mini brain' with great intelligence and power, which greatly influences our health and well-being.
- Our heart has its own nervous system, and can sense, learn, remember and make valuable decisions independent of the brain.
- Our heart sends messages to the brain and the rest of the body through hormones that influence our emotional reactions.
- Our heart communicates with and influences the head brain by way of the nervous system, the hormonal system and other nerve pathways. There is an ongoing two-way communication between the heart and brain, the one influencing the other's function.
- Our heart plays an important role in how we feel and think, and particularly in how we respond to stress.

Our emotions have a major impact on our heart

Every time our heart beats, it sends out powerful rhythmic signals and information to our head brain. These rhythms will either activate our stress response or a feeling of relaxation.

Specific heart rhythm patterns correspond to our different emotional states.

Negative emotions can cause our heart rhythms to become jagged – incoherent.

For example, if we **hold on** to stress or other negative emotions, such as anger, fear and frustration, we keep our heart rhythms chaotic and jagged. Stress hormones remain in our blood where they will cause damage.

Positive emotions create coherent heart rhythms. For example, love, gratitude, compassion, caring, joy and happiness promote smooth, harmonious heart rhythms. This brings relaxing hormones into our blood reducing our stress and creating feelings of well-being.

This gives us many remarkable benefits: a reduction in our blood pressure; a decrease in our stress hormones; a rise in our 'feel good factor' and anti-ageing hormone levels; a boost to our immune system.

Want to transform stress? – Alter your heart's rhythms

HeartMath's powerful tried and tested techniques enable you to regulate your own heart rhythms, alleviate stress and improve your overall health and well-being – mentally, emotionally and spiritually.

If you deliberately focus on your heart with positive feelings, such as love, appreciation, care or compassion, you can change your heart rhythms from chaotic and jagged rhythms into coherent ones.

Exercise 1   HeartMath 'Freeze Frame'

This exercise is an instant stress-buster that you can do anywhere and any time you are stressed. It is a one-minute powerful exercise that creates greater harmony in heart rhythms and reduces stress.

- It can help you to make a heartfelt shift in your perception and view stressful situations in a more hopeful light.
- If you tap into your heart's intelligence and intuitive ability, you may find a new creative solution to a stressful problem.
- It is a proven exercise for helping us to reach a clear decision by creating greater harmony between our heart and brain.
- This results in more efficient brain function.

Freeze Frame method

Pick one situation in the present that is stressing you. Spend a little time figuring out how this situation makes you think, feel and react. Now put all this on pause, as if you are putting a DVD on pause, and:

1 Place your hand over your heart. Shift your attention to the area of your heart and focus on your heart.

2 Do 'Heart Breathing'. Keep your focus on your heart by gently breathing – five seconds in and five seconds out – as if through the area of your heart. Do this two or three times.

3 Do 'Heart Feeling'. Recall one particular joyful or happy event in your life, or a specific time when you felt real appreciation or gratitude for someone or something in your life. Feel the real feelings of that memory as if you were actually there in the experience – living it – and hold on to those feelings.

4 Focus on that good heart feeling as you continue breathing through the area of your heart.

If you need to get a new perspective

1 Stay focused on the area around your heart.
  Ask your heart: 'What would be a better response to this situation in future? One that would cause less stress.' By asking this question from your heart with sincerity, your own intuition and good sense will be more available to you.

2 Stay relaxed and focused on your heart. Listen to the response of your heart.

As you listen to your heart, more often than not, you will experience some shift in perception or a creative insight into resolving the situation.

Whenever you find yourself challenged by life, that is the time to focus your awareness on your spiritual heart centre.

Ask it for the truth about yourself, others, and your situation.

Exercise 2 Simple 'Heart Lock-In'

This exercise will lock you in to smooth heart rhythms and will create a greater ability to hold onto positive emotions and feelings.

Heart Lock-Ins will enable you to develop the most important relationship of all – the relationship with yourself. They bring regenerative energy to your entire system and create a loving, open-hearted attitude.

Heart Lock-Ins will:

● Help to increase coherence within your heart and all your body's systems – mental, emotional, physical and spiritual.
● Tune you into your deeper loving heart, allowing you to respond to new energy.
● Increase your creativity and perceptiveness, willpower and inner security.
● It can increase your ability to love and develop compassion.

Heart Lock-In Method

1 Sit down in a comfortable place, close your eyes and relax.

2 Shift your attention away from your mind and focus on your heart area – place your hand on your heart. Imagine *breathing* in slowly through your heart and *breathing out* slowly through your solar plexus (an inch or two above your navel) for a short while.

3 Focus on a genuine feeling of appreciation or care you have for someone specific in your life – maybe a child, an adult or a pet. Or focus on a genuine feeling of appreciation for something positive you have in your life such as a beautiful garden or a park you love. Hold the image for a short time.

4 Then let go of the image – keep focused on those feelings of appreciation and care for 5–15 minutes.

5 Now send those feelings of love and appreciation to yourself and others.

6 If you notice your mind wandering, focus on breathing in through your heart and out through your solar plexus.

Important reminder No. 1
Chronic stress and a chronic pattern of holding onto negative emotions can put a great strain on your heart. It can raise your blood pressure and weaken your immune system.

Important reminder No. 2
Repeated stress and negative emotions disorder the heart's rhythms and the body's nervous system, damaging your health.

Important reminder No. 3
By creating heartfelt positive emotions, you will change your heart rhythms into smooth harmonious rhythms and bring relaxing and energising hormones into your blood, boosting your overall health and well-being.

Final Important reminder
A coherent heart rhythm has a positive effect on those around you. The reverse is also true — a jagged heart rhythm, called an incoherent heart rhythm, has a negative effect on those around you.

Heart-Lifting reminder

You can change your heart rhythms in the twinkling of an eye and bring relaxing and 'feel good factor' hormones into your blood.

17
Know Your Rights – Assert Yourself

Stand up for yourself – that is a must

'What has that to do with stress?' You may ask

'A whole load,' we would answer. Not being able to recognise our own rights and assert them is a major cause of stress and loss of confidence. It allows others to take advantage of us or treat us unfairly. It can cause us to miss out on many areas in our lives – including building a career; making good relationships; getting what we want and justly deserve. As a result, we can hold onto anger, hurt, pain and loss and be held back in life.

> Our personal human rights are those rights and expectations that all human beings have by virtue of our very existence.
>
> It is important to remember that other people have the same rights as we do and deserve respect and equally fair treatment.

Our basic personal human rights include:

- The right to **justice, respect** and **human dignity**
- The right to equal and fair treatment
- The right to live in or work in a secure, non-abusive environment
- The right to be in a non-abusive relationship

- The right to our own thoughts, opinions, feelings and values
- The right to express our opinions, thoughts, feelings and beliefs in an honest and open way that is respectful of others (great for improving relationships)
- The right to make mistakes and be responsible for them, realising that to make mistakes is part of being human and we can learn from them

- The right to ask for what we want and need while realising that the other person has the right to say 'No'
- The right to say 'No' to requests or demands that are unreasonable or that make us uncomfortable without having to give explanations
- The right to be independent and have interests of our own
- The right to make friends and be comfortable around people
- The right to determine and honour our own priorities

- The right to terminate conversations with others if they are being aggressive or abusive
- The right not to be responsible for another adult's behaviour, actions or problems
- The right to feel afraid, anxious, angry, upset or anything else and say so
- The right to look after all aspects of our health
- The right to forgive ourselves, learn the lesson and move on

What is assertiveness?

- It's the ability to know the true worth and value of ourselves and others, and to realise that we all deserve to be treated fairly and be happy.
- It's the ability to understand that others don't always feel or see things the same way as we do but deserve equal respect.
- It's about the ability to relate to others and communicate in an honest, open way with them.
- It's about being able to stand up for ourselves, resolve conflict with others and negotiate with them.

We need to be fully aware of our own rights and take into account that other people have the same rights as we have, and deserve equally fair treatment and respect.

We need to be aware that each of us is a unique human being, different yet equally valuable and deserving.

We can respect and value ourselves and others without comparing ourselves unfavourably with others – and build up our confidence and self-esteem.

Clear, honest communication is a must in being assertive

Clear, honest, open communication, including being able to express your feelings about a situation, is very important. Being clear about what you feel and what you want or need, and how it can be achieved, is also very important.

The 'I win and you win' solution is an assertive solution where the rights of both parties are recognised and respected and where both seek to reach a good compromise where possible.

No matter what the situation or problem is, people like to know that you respect them and want to work the situation out in a way that is best for both of you. This goes a long way towards resolving conflict and negotiating positive outcomes.

Portray your assertiveness with good body posture

Being assertive requires us to have a confident, open body posture, neither slumping nor victim-like. We need to respect our own space and that of others. It requires us to have good eye contact and a good tone of voice that is neither harsh nor accusing, nor weak and mumbling.

Being Assertive Means That:

- We engage with others in a respectful way; we stand up for our rights and do not allow others to abuse us, take advantage of us or treat us unfairly.
- We are able to talk openly about ourselves and can express our opinions, thoughts, feelings and beliefs directly, openly and honestly. We are able to listen to others and respect them.
- We are able to disagree and express positive or negative thoughts or feelings in a non-threatening way, and also be willing to receive positive and negative feedback.

- We are aware of what we want and we are able to ask for it in an open and direct way – and if we are refused we are not demolished. There are other options and solutions.
- We can take responsibility for our own decisions and actions.
- We can acknowledge our part in a conflict, resolve a conflict and negotiate a 'win-win' outcome for both ourselves and others.
- We have clear boundaries and can stick to them and defend our position with confidence, even if it provokes a conflict – and we are able to handle a conflict if it occurs.

Being assertive also means that we can acknowledge our strengths, recognise when we have done something well and accept a compliment – from ourselves and/or others.

18
Dealing With Confrontation

Stand up and be counted

> If you don't stand up for yourself, you leave yourself open to be taken advantage of or treated unfairly.
>
> Stand up for yourself and your confidence will increase.

Unfortunately, many people will treat you unfairly if you let them. Such people can include your boss, your work colleagues, your friends and even members of your own family. If you don't stand up for yourself nobody else can.

It is your own responsibility to stand up for yourself and prevent others treating you badly.

Many people are afraid of confrontation or avoid it, often telling themselves that nothing will change and that matters will only get worse. (That is most often caused by a childhood misguided belief.) **Being taken advantage of is not an option either for yourself or the other person involved.** You owe it to yourself to stand up for yourself.

Guidelines for confronting someone assertively

Don't be afraid of a bit of conflict – it is often necessary for fostering better relationships.

Asserting ourselves in an open, honest and direct way, without being unduly judgmental or critical of the other person, usually brings positive results.

Confronting another person can be difficult for some people. Therefore, if you make a plan as to how you are going to do it, you will feel more confident about doing it.

1 Your intentions will play a major part in how successful the outcome will be. It's important that, firstly, you are clear yourself about *why* you intend to confront the other person. For example, do you want them to *stop doing* something? Do you want to *resolve* some conflict with them? Or do you just want a great big fight?

2 Ask yourself, 'What exactly have they done, are doing or not doing, as the case may be, that is bothering me? Is there something I want them to stop doing because it is unfair to me? What do I want them to do instead?'
   If you are being treated unfairly, for example, be clear as to *when*, *where* and *how*. How often does it happen? Where does it happen? What is it in the behaviour of the other person that makes you feel they are treating you unfairly?

3 Ask yourself, 'What part, if any, do I play in this situation?' Think about it – be honest with yourself.

4 Plan ahead. Decide exactly what you are going to say and when would be the most opportune time. Request a time with the other person, telling them you want to talk to them about something that is bothering you. Timing is important – don't wait till they are drunk or in a rush!

5 Keep your communication straightforward, honest and to the point. *Say exactly what they are doing that is upsetting you* – and the *reason it upsets you* and *how it affects you emotionally*. Give them example/s of when, where and how this happens.

6 Say clearly *what you want to happen* instead.

7 Negotiate an agreement with them and resolve problems where necessary.

One illustrative scenario – Tony and his boss, Jason

This model can be used or applied in most situations:

Susan, a work colleague of Tony's has been off sick for the past two weeks. They work together in a very busy department where they have deadlines to meet. Since Susan went off sick, Jason, the boss, has left Susan's workload on Tony's desk for Tony to complete on top of his own.

1 **Identify the unacceptable behaviour**
   Tony to Jason: 'For the past two weeks, since Susan has been off sick from work, you have left a pile of Susan's work on my desk for me to deal with as well as my own.'

2 **Identify the consequences**
   Tony to Jason: 'I am already under pressure to get my own work done. I now have a backlog of my own work as well as most of Susan's, both of which are impossible to complete now. On top of that, I am pressured by my two supervisors who are stressed and demanding because I haven't had time to get this report ready for them.'

3 **Express how you feel**
   Tony to Jason: 'I feel cross and unfairly put upon. I feel that expecting me to do Susan's work as well as my own is unrealistic and unfair – I work to deadlines already and am very busy.'

4 **Own up to your responsibility – (Tony has contributed to the problems caused by Susan's absence)**
   Tony admitted to himself and his boss the part he played in the situation and said that, in hindsight, he could have discussed and resolved the problem with Jason two weeks ago – the day Jason first left him Susan's first workload. (Then Jason would have had to find a better solution to the problem and Tony would not have felt put upon!)

5 **Express what you want to happen**
   Tony to Jason: 'It's important now that we resolve this situation. I would like you to make other arrangements as of now regarding Susan's work because I am unable to do it. So here it is [Tony hands Susan's work back to Jason] – I have put the sections I have done in the green folder.'

Let the other person express themselves but not veer off the point, and if they do, bring it back to the problem, saying 'I want this resolved now – we can address the other topics later.' (Tony cannot let Jason spin any hard-luck story or put pressure on him – he needs to stick to his guns.)

6 **Negotiate a resolution if needed – perhaps negotiate a win-win situation for both of you**

Tony to Jason: 'I am willing to work paid overtime just for the next few days to catch up with the backlog of my own work. This will relieve some of the pressure on me and my department.'

It is very common for people who have a non-assertive pattern to justify why things will either get worse or nothing will change if they assert themselves.

This type of thinking is usually fuelled by a misguided subconscious belief from childhood.

19
Understand Your Emotions

We are emotional beings

Our emotions are fundamental to who we are.

If we don't learn to deal with them in a helpful way, we shall open ourselves up to a lot of stress and unhappiness.

We wouldn't be able to think or function properly without our emotions. If we felt no sadness, no fear, no regret, no anger, no guilt, no joy, no love, we would be like robots, unable to feel empathy or compassion. We would be unable to evolve.

How we can grow emotionally

We need to acknowledge our own emotions and allow ourselves to *experience them* and *express them safely*. We need to try and understand what message they are giving us. For example, if we feel very angry we need to understand why we are angry and who we are angry with and for what reason. We need to discharge this anger. Perhaps we need to have a good old rant or cry or talk to someone (perhaps acknowledge what part we played in the situation, if any) and resolve conflict with the person we are angry with. When we do this we develop emotionally and increase our self-confidence and self-worth. Our relationships will improve and become more meaningful. We, ourselves, will become more carefree, joyful and happy.

How do we bury painful emotions?

Our culture does not encourage us to express our emotions so, to our detriment, we often bury painful emotions.

- We may hide from our painful emotions because we don't want to experience pain, be that pain from fear, grief, anger, guilt, shame, self-blame or humiliation.
- We may dismiss our emotions by minimising what has happened to us.
- We may feel that showing our emotions is not acceptable – we may be afraid that we shall be judged harshly.
- We may just plain ignore them.

What happens when we don't deal with our painful emotions?

- If we don't deal with our strong negative emotions, we are stuck in them and we might experience them, one way or another, over and over again, creating misery and unhappiness for ourselves.

- We may experience underlying anxiety, end up sulking, feeling resentful, hard done by or victimised.

- We may find ourselves getting angry or over-critical in response to minor slights, and behave badly towards others.

- Our painful buried emotions can be re-awakened and re-experienced in the present. This can happen as a result of any interaction or situation that reminds us of the original situation that caused us to bury them. Then our emotional reactions to present-day situations can be out of all proportion to what is actually happening.

- If we have a pattern of not dealing with negative emotions, they will have a very negative effect on our relationships, particularly on those people close to us, because nothing much can be resolved and the same problems will recur.

- If we bury our strong negative emotions, they can get stuck in our muscles, ligaments, and other parts of the body, where they can distort or block our energy.

Important reminder No. 1

Realise that you are not alone. Burying strong negative emotions is very common. If you have a lot of unresolved painful emotions, it might be good to seek short-term professional help to deal with them.

Important reminder No. 2

If you have a lot of unresolved negative emotions, your emotional reactions in the present may not always be in proportion to what is actually happening.

Important reminder No. 3

Dump not your unresolved emotions on the undeserving! Not only can it make them feel bad, it can make you feel bad, too.

The most important reminder

If you release your painful emotions, you will become more honest with yourself and others, more confident and more courageous.

20
Increase Your Emotional Intelligence

Advance your emotional intelligence and gain a better life

If you have worked through some of the chapters in this book, you will already have increased your emotional intelligence along the way.

Gaining more emotional intelligence will enable you to live a much happier, more peaceful life.

Emotional intelligence is important for good health and well-being.

It is essential for self-development and developing good relationships with others.

Emotional intelligence includes having the ability to:

- Recognise and understand your emotions
- Control and manage your emotions
- Manage your behaviour
- Understand your needs
- Be aware of others' emotions and their needs
- Have empathy and put yourself in another's shoes
- Take care of every aspect of your health and well-being

Some tips for improving your emotional intelligence

Become more aware of what *triggers* your stress reaction and recognise how it affects your body, including your breathing, your mind and your emotions.

- Examine your thoughts, perceptions and behaviours in these situations. For example, do you get anxious when you make a simple mistake? Do you become angry or upset every time something doesn't happen the way you want? Do you blame others or become angry with them, even when it's not their fault?

- Gain control of your own emotions and knee-jerk reactions so that you can weigh up situations and respond with a balanced reaction to what is happening. Express your emotions in a helpful way.

- Understand others better and develop *Empathy*. This is a very important part of developing emotional intelligence. Empathy is the ability to recognise and understand the feelings, wants, needs and viewpoints of those around you (without being too judgmental or harsh). Metaphorically speaking, it is the ability to put ourselves in another's shoes. This is a must for developing fairness and compassion.

- Begin to recognise how your reactions and behaviour may affect others and become more aware of how others may perceive you.

- Express regret if you have distressed others unduly and learn from it.

- Take responsibility for yourself, your own behaviour and actions. Develop the courage to look at yourself honestly, recognise unhelpful behaviours in yourself, and make an effort to change them.

- Get to know your strengths and weaknesses, and work to improve your weaknesses and appreciate your strengths.

- Learn to motivate yourself and take on new challenges and develop your own talents and creative abilities.

Get a lot more out of your life

By developing your emotional intelligence you will be able to give time, energy and commitment to your needs. This is essential for developing and maintaining good health and for living a happier life!

Some important skills for developing emotional intelligence

- Stress control and management
- Good honest, open communication

- The art of negotiation, conflict resolution and anger management
- Assertiveness which takes into account other people's rights as well as your own
- Problem-solving
- Prioritising and goal-setting
- Fostering good honest relations with others

Now read, enjoy and ponder the following metaphorical story

Black Stripe Across The Red Bottoms

'I can't help it if I'm the only monkey that has a white fluffy bottom,' said Jadpour the monkey. He was sick and tired of the other monkeys laughing at him and taunting him because he did not have a big red bottom that flashed like theirs.

Jadpour had no peace at all: if it wasn't one monkey, it was another who would march up to him, stand in front of him and flash a big red bottom at him. The monkeys seemed to flash their bottoms incessantly – from the time they woke up in the morning until the time they went to bed. They were always irritable and frazzled from all the bottom-flashing and had little time for anything else.

One day, Jadpour told the taunting monkeys, 'I have golden soft hair like the sun on my chest.'

That was a particularly bad day for Jadpour. Each monkey was enraged at Jadpour's proud declaration about his golden soft chest hair. One by one, they came over to him and bit him hard, drawing blood.

All the other monkeys had brown, rough 'wire brush' hair on their chests that pricked their hands when they scratched themselves.

At night, all the monkeys slept in the big monkey nest high up in the tallest tree in the rainforest. Jadpour was never allowed into the monkey nest because he didn't have a flashing red bottom; instead, he had to sleep alone in the small nest that he had made for himself nearby.

One night, when the moon was big and Jadpour couldn't sleep, he stole away to the distant forest where the Hoc Hoc tree grew. The Hoc Hoc tree gladly gave Jadpour a pot of her black indelible ink-dye. When Jadpour got home, all the monkeys were still fast asleep in their big monkey nest. They were snoring loudly. They had all eaten the sleep-inducing fruit of the Sa Sa tree and were unlikely to wake up before midday.

With the ink of the Hoc Hoc tree, Jadpour painted a big black stripe right across each of the monkeys' red flashing bottoms. The monkeys never woke up during the delicate task of painting the black stripe.

At midday, when the monkeys woke up and discovered the black stripe on their once flashing red bottoms, they were beside themselves. They jumped about, beating their chests, hollering, stamping their feet, roaring, screaming and growling. They were confused and enraged.

Jadpour calmly watched them from the safety of a nearby tree where he sat eating a banana and a handful of nuts.

The screaming and chest-beating and roaring went on for seven whole days and nights. On the eighth day, a great hush and calm came over the monkeys. They sat in pure silence and stillness for hours. Jadpour watched from a safe distance.

Suddenly, a big alpha male monkey got up and announced to all that they needed to collect fruit and nuts and other delicacies for a great feast.

Each monkey collected a stash of food and carried it to a grassy spot near their big tree. Soon there was enough food for a great feast.

Jadpour, too, collected food and kept his in a little pile a safe distance from the rest of the monkeys. Towards evening, they all gathered round to enjoy the food feast.

A big old alpha male monkey walked slowly over to where Jadpour sat, alone and confused. He told him to pick up his food and come over to join the feast with the rest of the monkeys. One by one, each monkey came over to greet Jadpour and rub his head affectionately.

The old alpha male monkey made a speech. 'We are celebrating this evening the remarkable magic arrival of the black stripe across our bottoms. We are now happy that we no longer need to flash our bottoms – this is a great and true blessing – a great release. Now we have more time to play and groom and rest and dream and explore the forest – truly, a miracle has taken place.'

That night, all the monkeys, including Jadpour, slept together, cosy and safe, in the big monkey nest on top of the tallest tree.

21
Carry Not The Bag Of Resentment

How heavy is your bag of resentment?

If your bag of resentment is heavy, you don't have to carry it around with you and that can only be good news.

If we carry a bag of resentment with us, we shall re-experience painful events and emotions over and over again. This will have a very negative, destructive effect on us psychologically – mentally, emotionally, physically and spiritually.

Resentment is a very common feeling that we as human beings experience. We can harbour resentment when we feel people have hurt or abused or taken advantage of us in some way. We can also store up resentment when people don't match up to our expectations of them.

When we **hold onto** resentment, we hold a ball of hurt and anger inside our hearts. We can become bitter and nurse the old hurts for a long time, even a lifetime.

Holding onto resentment may be a family pattern we are living out – we may need to realise this before we are able to let go. Also, we may live in continuous resentment because we confuse people in the present with people in the past who have hurt or rejected us in some way.

The sad thing about resentment, however justified it may be, is that the person who holds onto resentment and bitterness is the one who will continue to suffer.

Think about it: the person who has hurt or treated us badly probably isn't bothered by it or is often oblivious of the fact that we resent them.

Bitterness and resentment, if held onto, can take over our lives and destroy our joy and happiness.

How we deal with hurt or unfairness will play a big part in how happy we are in life.

If we deal with hurt in a helpful way, we shall bring joy into our hearts and not grow resentful.

Life is full of ups and downs

Yes, it's a fact of life – people hurt each other. Either intentionally or unintentionally, we shall hurt each other because we are imperfect human beings. The reality is that we are going to hurt people at times and they are going to hurt us – and that is how life goes. Many things that happen to us in life are not fair but that is how life is – that is how the cookie crumbles!

Letting go of resentment is a good choice

Letting go of resentment is a choice we make. Often we don't know how to let go of hurt, anger, feelings of rejection and other painful feelings (if this is the case, it may be advisable to seek professional help). Long-term resentment can create insecurity and depression.

Often as humans we may have difficulty acknowledging the part we played in creating the problem – if we indeed had a part to play. If we really don't want to acknowledge our part, we are giving ourselves a licence to be self-righteous and hold onto resentment.

Stand up for yourself – hints don't work!

Since we all feel differently and often perceive things differently, sometimes the people we resent don't even know how or what we are really feeling. We think that we are giving them enough *hints* and *signs* and they should know how we feel.

Whenever possible, if someone has hurt you or treated you badly, you need to stand up for yourself and be totally truthful and honest with them. Tell them what they have done to hurt you and what exactly you feel about that. Being able to resolve a problem with another person – when possible – will allow you to let go of painful emotions.

Forgiveness sets us free

When we forgive, we are able to let go of resentment, grudges, bitterness and the desire to retaliate. Forgiveness can bring you peace and emotional healing – it frees you up to be yourself again and breaks the power the other person has in your life.

> Forgiveness is not about denying the other person's responsibility for hurting you or minimising the wrong they did to you.
>
> The pain and hurt caused to you may remain part of your life.
>
> Forgiveness is the gift to yourself that will weaken the hold resentment and bitterness have over you.

Holding onto resentment is like holding a time bomb

Long-term deep resentment is a self-destructive force. It can take away our peace of mind because it prolongs our hurt and so make us miserable. It can constantly generate feelings of anger, shame and rage and make us feel hard done by. It can make us depressed, stressed, despairing and self-obsessed and have us wallowing in self-pity. It can affect our personality, driving us to seek more causes of resentment, going from one to the next.

Resentment can hurt our physical health and relationships

It can keep us stressed and play havoc with our health, damaging our vital organs and our immune system, which is the body's natural defence against disease. It makes us very negative and inclined to focus on what we haven't got, rather than on all that we already have.

Bitterness and resentment can make us develop a hypercritical attitude and grumpiness towards those around us. It can make others want to avoid us and then we may feel rejected and more bitter. We can get angry quickly and then resentful when things don't go our way.

Free yourself first by forgiving yourself

Forgiving ourselves allows us to release old feelings of fear, shame, guilt and anger against ourselves.

Just as it is more difficult to love others if we don't love ourselves also, it is much harder to forgive others if we don't forgive ourselves.

When we are able to forgive ourselves, we are able to let go of that little destructive part of ourselves that wants to control us. We need to accept that we are imperfect human beings and that, at times, like everyone else, we shall mess up in one way or another. Lack of forgiveness can keep us dwelling on the past, beating ourselves up for what we did or didn't do. It can stop us living happily in the present and make us fear the future.

How to forgive yourself

- Acknowledge the events in your life that make you feel bad and guilty.
- Thank your spirit for allowing you to see them clearly and acknowledge them.
- If there is something you can do about what is causing you to feel bad, be brave and do it.
- If you are beating yourself up for something that you did or didn't do, learn the lesson – if there is nothing you can do, forgive yourself and move on.
- If you have hurt someone, acknowledge it, ask their forgiveness and move on.

Exercise in forgiving yourself and others

Realise you are a beautiful, unique, lovable human being and can now forgive yourself, learn and grow.

Spend a few moments indentifying any resentments you may hold.

Make a quick list of them and then choose one from your list. (You can gradually work through your own list.)

Sit down where you are comfortable and won't be disturbed.

- Take some relaxing breaths first.
- Imagine that you have a big old bag of resentment strapped to your back which represents the resentment you want to work on. This bag may well contain a lot of guilt, self-blame and negative emotions that you have been holding against yourself or others.
- The bag feels heavy and uncomfortable on your back.
- The rough black material feels prickly against your skin.
- It smells awful – just like sour overripe cheese and it makes you feel nauseous.
- There is a sloshing noise coming from the bag as though something were splashing around inside it.

- You spot a bright fire close by and realise that you don't have to carry this horrible burden around on your back any more.
- You prise the bag from your back and dump it into the heart of the fire.
- You watch as it is quickly consumed by the flames of the burning fire.

- You breathe a sigh of relief, shake your shoulders out and stand tall.
- Now spend a little time sending love and gratitude to your heart.

Repeat this exercise as often as is necessary and more frequently if you have this pattern.

22
A View On Spirituality

A brief take on spirituality

We don't profess to be any authority on spirituality – it's hard to imagine that anyone really is. Spirituality has a different meaning for different people and this is just one take on it.

Spirituality is not necessarily about a particular religion or creed, although religion may be a way of expressing your spirituality.

Maybe love is the key to our happiness

Developing our spirituality can help us gain access to our inner wisdom, the truth and knowledge that are part of who we are.

Access to this truth and wisdom allows us to develop greater love and compassion for ourselves, for others, and for our planet.

To function fully as human beings, all aspects of ourselves – mind, body, emotions and spirit – need to be in balance.

The need for spirituality in our daily lives

Spirituality needs to be practised in our daily lives if it is to mean anything. Developing spiritually is about striving to cultivate the noblest qualities of our human spirit, rather than always following the drives of self-gratification and materialism.

It means that we continue to strive to develop love, empathy, compassion, courage, honesty, equality, freedom and generosity. Then we shall be more able to forgive ourselves and others and develop a deeper sense of responsibility towards each other and our planet.

Our connection to all

As we develop spiritually, we become less entrenched in the drives of our ego – less selfish – and our hunger for power, recognition and social status will become less important in our lives. They will be replaced by giving and sharing with others. This is maybe where our true freedom and joy lie.

Evolving spiritually can help us deepen a spirit of gratitude, co-operation and connection to others, whereby we help each other – friend and stranger. This gives us a sense of peace, contentment, comradeship and connectedness with our fellow human beings. The barrier between ourselves and others will begin to crumble, giving us a deeper connection to, and compassion for, ourselves and others, and indeed the whole planet.

It seems that a need for these qualities is rooted in the core of our being and gives us comfort, strength, happiness and joy. The more we evolve spiritually, the more loving, joyful, giving and generous we become.

By fostering our connection to nature, the earth and the planet, we renew ourselves with the inspiring majesty, wonder and beauty of all life. This connection nourishes our spirit, giving us a greater perspective on life.

Any practice that quells our racing minds – like being out in nature, meditating, healing imagery, healing visualizations, HeartMath, listening to tranquil music, or painting – brings us closer to our authentic self – our spirit. This is why these practices are regarded as giving nourishment to our spirit.

You need to find regular times throughout the day to still your busy mind and get in touch with your inner wisdom and spirit.

Spirituality fosters inner security

The closer we get to our true spiritual self, the freer we become from our fears and insecurities. We can find an inner peace and security and happiness that do not always depend on external things or circumstances.

Ignoring our spiritual side can leave us feeling isolated, lonely and dissatisfied with life. We can miss out on the everyday joys of living while chasing our next 'fix'.

An exercise to foster a deeper connection to your 'spirit-self'

This exercise helps us to realise that we are not just our physical bodies, emotions, thoughts, desires, or attitudes. We are a centre of pure consciousness – our spirit-self.

(This exercise is based on a Psychosynthesis approach to psychology developed by Roberto Assagioli M.D.)

If you do this exercise frequently, you will become more aware of your own true nature, your true essence.

Sit down quietly where you won't be disturbed.

Just become aware of your body.

- Just for a few moments, be objective – don't try to change anything, just observe.
- Be aware of how you are breathing – whether fast, shallow, slowly or deeply – whether through your nose or mouth.
- Become aware of your posture and how you are sitting – upright or slumped.
- Be aware of the contact of your body with the chair and your feet with the floor.
- Become aware of any physical sensations in your body, such as pain, tension, tightness, tenderness or soreness. Notice whether or not you are comfortable, relaxed and calm, or hot and sweaty, or cold.

Become aware of your feelings.

- Just observe your feelings neutrally and don't try to change anything – just observe.
- What kind of feelings are you experiencing right now? Are you happy and contented, or sad, insecure and lonely, or resentful and angry?

Turn to your desires now.

- Just observe your desires – again neutrally – and don't try to change anything, just observe.
- Become aware of the chief desires which motivate your life, such as a desire for love, or a successful career, or fame and fortune.

Turn your attention to your thoughts.

- Just observe your thoughts neutrally – without any judgement. Don't try to change anything – just observe.
- As soon as a thought emerges, observe it until another one takes its place, do the same with the next and the next and so on.
- Observe your stream of consciousness as it flows by – memories, opinions, 'mind- chatter', comments, judgments, arguments, images.
- Do this for a couple of minutes, then stop observing and

Q: Ask yourself – Who is it that has been doing all this observing?
A: Could it be my spirit-self – my true essence – my higher self?

Consider this for a few moments:

'You' are not your thoughts. You are not an image or a thought or an emotion or a desire. Your spirit-self has been observing all these. You are that being.

23
Self-Esteem – Your Key To A Happier Life

Our self-esteem and our happiness are closely intertwined

Our self-esteem is at the root of our personal power, our inner security, what we believe we are capable of and how deserving and worthy we feel.

Our self-esteem is very important in our lives because it affects our whole life and how we live it.

Let's look at what self-esteem is about

Self-esteem is how we really feel about ourselves. It's about:

- The type of person we believe we are.
- How important, equal, worthwhile and good we believe we are.
- How worthy, valuable and deserving of love and respect we feel.
- How much power and capability we believe we have.

Now that you have gained some good skills and resources, you will also have increased your self-esteem somewhat. Why not develop even greater and more robust self-esteem?

Good robust self-esteem will enable you to:

- Have a good opinion of yourself, respect yourself, feel that you are an equally valuable, worthwhile person, deserving of happiness and equality like everyone else.

- Be able to like, love, appreciate and accept yourself – flaws and all – and be your own best friend through the ups and downs of life.

- Be able to recognise and appreciate your own good qualities, your past achievements, and your strengths and capabilities and build on them. (Your greatest achievement might be about surviving a bad time and not carrying a bag of resentment with you, or sharing with others what you want to keep yourself or learning to get along with people better – your achievements are as vast and varied as are your qualities and capabilities.)

- Be able to acknowledge and accept your own weaknesses without comparing yourself unfavourably with others or judging yourself too harshly.

- Want to strive to strengthen your weaknesses, acknowledge your mistakes, and when you make them, learn from them, forgive yourself and others and move on.

- Be better able to face life's challenges, exercise your own power and stand up for yourself.

- Be able to develop your capabilities and enjoy life more.

Good self-esteem is essential for developing a confident, positive and hopeful attitude towards life, for being more resourceful in life and for being able to live life to the full.

If you have good self-esteem, you will want to treat others with equal respect, fairness, kindness and generosity and you will be able to ask for help and support yourself when you need it.

Get good self-esteem and get the best from your life

Good self-esteem will make you proud to be who you are and realise that you deserve joy and happiness in life. You will be better able to make good choices and decisions for yourself and have the courage to meet and deal with life's challenges in the best way.

Good self-esteem will enable you to take more responsibility for yourself and know that you have the power and ability to learn, grow and achieve many things in life.

You will feel more determined to take better care of all aspects of your health and happiness, develop self-sufficiency and contribute to the world around you.

A negative opinion of yourself sells yourself short

Low self-esteem can negatively influence almost every aspect of your life, including your confidence, happiness, your relationships and the kinds of choices you make.

A negative view of yourself can leave you feeling anxious, self-critical, and often powerless and low, with poor resistance to stress. It may leave you over-reliant on the opinions and reactions of others to determine your self-worth.

Very few people are without some dents in their self-esteem

Some of us will have less self-esteem than others. Even those who appear to have good self-esteem, may battle underneath the surface with feelings of worthlessness. Most people would say that they could do with a boost to their self-esteem!

Our self-esteem is shaped by our unconscious beliefs

Our self-esteem comes from the beliefs we hold about ourselves in our unconscious mind.

If we carry *untruthful beliefs* about ourselves, they have a powerful negative impact on our self-esteem and can override our rational selves.

If, for example, you erroneously believe that you are not as capable as others, it won't matter how capable you are or what you have achieved, your unconscious belief will still pop up at times, flooding you with self-doubt.

Negative unconscious beliefs about ourselves will continue to damage us if we don't change them.

How much these beliefs affect you will depend on how strong they are and how much you feed into them.

Before we show you how to build up really strong self-esteem, you need first to understand a little about these unconscious beliefs that hold the key to your self-esteem. You can learn all about them in the following chapter.

24
Our Unconscious Beliefs

Our unconscious beliefs, our powerhouse

Our unconscious beliefs are the powerhouse of our self-esteem and stress levels

Your unconscious beliefs captain your ship

Your unconscious beliefs have a huge influence on how you live your daily life. They tell you how to think, feel and behave. They tell you how to feel about yourself and others, how to relate to yourself and others and the world at large.

Each of us has our own beliefs, attitudes and views and these make us unique.

Most of our beliefs operate outside our conscious awareness and seem so normal to us that we don't even question them, yet they profoundly affect our whole life.

Your thoughts, views, feelings, attitudes and behaviours flow from your unconscious beliefs. These act as internal guides, telling you how to think about each situation you encounter, how to interpret it, how to feel about it and how to react to it.

Your childhood – the birthplace of your beliefs

Your unconscious mind is the keeper of all you have ever experienced – the good and bad; everything you have seen, heard or done; everything you have learned, including your past impressions and associations; everything you have lived through; all your emotions, memories, reactions and behaviours.

As a young child, you were like a little sponge absorbing everything from your environment. You absorbed everything you experienced, every message you received, positive and negative, and every piece of information or misinformation.

From the way in which you understood and gave meaning to your childhood experiences, and the information and messages you received, you formed your own beliefs.

Although you may have changed, updated or deleted some of these original beliefs, many of them are still very alive and active today and they still guide and direct you. They still let you know how to view each of your present-day experiences, how to feel about them and how to react and deal with them.

Over the years, your beliefs become stronger and more deeply rooted, causing you to repeat the same patterns of response to your experiences, often making you feel miserable, angry or stressed. They have been with you so long that you believe in their truth.

Childhood beliefs – a child's perception

It's important to know that many of the beliefs that cause us the most stress are not always based on truth, but on a perception of what we as children understood as truth.

Many of these beliefs are simply the conclusions that we as small children came to, based on our limited understanding.

Our ability to rationalise was not even developed at the time.

Many of our unconscious beliefs are very helpful and positive and have a good impact on our lives. They support us and help us to deal with the ups and downs of life in the best possible way.

Unfortunately, most of us have some unhelpful, untruthful beliefs that distort our view of ourselves and make us feel less worthy than we really are.

The hardest hitters – our childhood's untrue core beliefs

> Most of our painful experiences and high stress levels spring from the deepest untruthful beliefs and assumptions that we hold about ourselves and our own identity.
>
> These beliefs are often called our Core Beliefs because they are at the core of our identity and self-esteem.

Our Core Beliefs have the most impact on us because they are at the root of our confidence and self-esteem. They tell us how to feel about ourselves. They form the basic assumptions we make about how lovable, equally valuable and worthwhile we are; how capable we believe we are; how much security we imagine we have; and how much personal power we think we have.

As a young child, you learned how to *feel* about yourself, about others, and the world around you through the actions and responses of parents, teachers and other important adults in your life (as well as siblings).

Your **emotionally distressing** negative experiences, such as repeated negative criticism, put-downs, or unfavourable comparisons may have caused you to form some flawed core beliefs about yourself.

This is the really good part

When you *change*, or *even dilute*, one major **untrue core belief**, your self-esteem and confidence will benefit from a major boost and many things in your life will change for the better.

Remember, most of your **untrue core beliefs** were never yours in the first place but imposed on you as a child. Why should you live your life carrying the false belief that other people are better than you - more lovable than you - more deserving than you - more powerful than you - more capable than you?

You are unique and have your own resources, talents and abilities and you have myriad possibilities waiting to be tapped. Your whole life is a learning experience and, like a river flowing to the sea, you don't want to be held back by the wreckage of your childhood's **untrue core beliefs**.

We are in this belief thing together

All of us as human beings have some **untrue core beliefs** about ourselves – you are not alone in this. The negative impact that they will have on your life depends on how strong the beliefs are and how much you feed into them.

A childhood **untrue core belief** can often lie sleeping until it is triggered by a particular life experience which resonates with the earlier experience that caused the initial imprinting. When this happens, we are often left feeling anxious and really doubting ourselves.

Untrue core beliefs can for some of us manifest themselves as an inflated ego – a false self-image which can lead to delusions of superiority and entitlement, and forgetting our common humanity and connection to each other and all life. We are all equally special. Our **untrue core beliefs** can foster unbridled greed, selfishness and extensive manipulation while smothering our compassion.

Without a doubt, our **untrue core beliefs** have the ability to make us feel unduly anxious and powerless, underestimate our ability, criticise and condemn ourselves all too readily. They will keep us operating below par, constantly sabotage our confidence and self-esteem, and trap us in a stressful life.

Our excellent skills and techniques in Resource 4 in Part Two will help you build super, robust self-esteem. They will enable you to:

- Identify your **untrue core beliefs**
- Weaken and change them
- Take on board your **true core beliefs** which will enable you to realise your own true value and worth and understand how capable and powerful you really are!

PART TWO

Resources

Resource 1
Identify Your Cognitive Distortions

Do we all have cognitive distortions?

We all have at least some cognitive distortions (irrational thinking patterns) which cause us to think in unhelpful rigid ways and that distort our view of reality. The degree to which you have them will determine how much they negatively affect your life. The reason we hold onto them is because we don't recognise them in ourselves – to us, they appear to be normal ways of thinking.

Now the good news! You can free yourself from your cognitive distortions.

This is your chance now to spot some in yourself.

We shall show you how to recognise some of the most common ones that can warp your view of yourself, others and situations that leave you at times feeling angry, upset, or hard done by, and stressed.

If they don't stress you, they may well be stressing others!

Have fun – check out your common cognitive distortions

From the list and information below, you can check and see if you can spot any cognitive distortions that might be very familiar to you.

Exercise to identify your own cognitive distortions

First, read through the following list of **Nine Common Cognitive Distortions** slowly, pondering each one.

See if you recognise any of these repetitive patterns in yourself.

If you do, tick off the pattern and write it down – you can work on it later.

No. 1   A pattern of black and white thinking – you view many things as either black or white

Are you seeing the full picture or just a little part of it?

This view causes us to think in extreme ways and as a result we can miss the full picture – we see part of the picture instead of the whole. We view events, ourselves and people as right or wrong, good or bad, black or white – there are no shades of grey.

Someone is either good or bad, stupid or clever. We may see our own endeavours or others' endeavours as successes or complete failures – nothing in-between. We may see situations as bad or good – nothing in-between.

We may tend to focus on what is happening from a negative viewpoint. We may wrongly assume that others think in extreme ways too, and we may feel they either like us or they really dislike us.

Some things really are black and white and that is fine; however, we need to understand and acknowledge that most life experiences and most people are not all good or all bad but contain elements of both.

> This particular pattern can promote a critical and judgmental attitude towards others and often ourselves – it can really mess up relationships.

No. 2 A pattern of catastrophic thinking – a tendency to assume the worst

Are you seeing things in proportion to what is actually happening or likely to happen??? Most of us are familiar with this one!

This one is a great anxiety-maker. With this thinking pattern, we can blow minor events out of proportion and exaggerate the negative aspects and consequences of past, present or future events.

We predict disasters that are, in fact, unlikely to occur and jump from one crisis to another. We focus on the worst possible outcome, however far-fetched, or think that a situation is intolerable when, in reality, it is just uncomfortable. We can drive ourselves mad and others, too!

Of course, there will be some life events that will cause us anxiety. However, most everyday events are part and parcel of life and do not call for a 'catastrophic' reaction.

This way of thinking can make us feel unnecessarily anxious and fearful, wasting our precious energy and time.

No. 3 A pattern of over-sensitivity and jumping to wrong conclusions

Are you over-sensitive and imagining insult where none is intended or jumping to the wrong conclusions?

With this pattern, we make decisions and arguments based on how we feel, rather than on the reality. If we let ourselves be caught up in this type of emotional reasoning, we can be misled by our feelings and confuse them with facts.

We can be over-sensitive and defensive, hurt or angry, and feel misjudged or undermined by the slightest perceived criticism. We can misinterpret others' intentions without any real evidence.

We wrongly assume that our distress is a result of others' behaviour when it may not necessarily be so. We assume that everything people say or do, or whatever mood they are in, is somehow related to us or is a reaction to us.

We can come to conclusions, usually negative, with little evidence to back them up. We can assume we know others' thoughts or intentions and predict how things will turn out like some crazed guru!

Being upset or angry if someone unjustly and harshly criticises us or hurts us is normal. However, people can say things that they themselves wouldn't consider hurtful. They may even like you and bear you no malice. It's important to remember that people have different ways of communicating.

In this cognitive distortion, we can take one or two isolated negative experiences and assume that all other related experiences will be the same. For example, if we fail one exam, we may conclude that we are no good at exams and a failure.

We can exaggerate the frequency of problems and jump to the wrong conclusions. For example, if someone is angry with us once, our conclusion may be 'This person is always angry with me' or 'He/she is just an angry person.' This distortion truly affects our view of ourselves and others, knocks our confidence and damages our relationships with people.

This pattern can inhibit others from being open and honest with us, even those who care about us the most.

It can cause us no end of distress and leave us feeling victimised without reason.

It can damage relationships – people may feel that they are perpetually treading on egg-shells!

Do we really know what someone else is thinking or feeling?

It is a good idea to give the person involved the benefit of the doubt until we have real proof that it is otherwise.

No. 4 A pattern of guilt and self-blame

Do you carry unnecessary guilt or blame yourself unjustly?

With this pattern, we tend to personalise everything and hold ourselves to blame for events that are not under our control. For example, your son takes off with a wayward woman and you tell yourself, 'It must be all my fault. If I had been a better mother to him, this would not have happened.'

We can blame ourselves entirely for things that are not all our fault, rather than taking responsibility for just our part in them. We may even blame ourselves for something that we have no part in at all.

We may blame ourselves for not being perfect and beat ourselves up for having made a mistake.

We may never allow ourselves to forget a mistake, forgive, learn the lesson and move on.

Do you think that a past mistake should be held over your head for the rest of your life or are you expecting yourself to be perfect?

No. 5   A pattern of blaming others and avoiding responsibility

Do you blame others and avoid responsibility for your share?

This is a very common cognitive distortion that we observe in many people.

In this pattern, we can hold other people responsible for our distress. For example, we may use phrases like 'Stop making me feel bad about myself!' Once we realise that we, and we alone, have control over our emotional reactions, we shall feel a lot better.

This pattern can mean blaming others for upsetting situations that we played a big part in or avoiding responsibility for our part. We may even try dumping responsibility onto others. We may even twist the situation around to make ourselves the injured party. We may unconsciously deny what is 'really happening' by refusing to talk about it.

Are you able to recognise and take responsibility for the part you play in situations?

We all need to take responsibility for our actions. However, it's important to understand that making mistakes is part of the human condition and is often an important way of learning and evolving. When we are able to hold up our hands to our mistakes, we feel much better about ourselves.

> Unless we take responsibility for our own actions and behaviour, we shall always be stuck in self-sabotaging behaviour and stress.

No. 6   A pattern of being addicted to work?

Do you overwork just to prove yourself to others and to feel valued?

Our work performance is linked to how we value ourselves. The pattern of being addicted to work can mean that work takes priority over everything in our life. Even when we are away from it, we think about it and we are obsessed with it – work is our life! We can neglect our relationships, health and well-being. We may have unrealistic expectations of how much others should work and put undue pressure on them.

There is nothing wrong with working hard, doing a good job and feeling valued for that. However, it's important to remember that there is more to life and living than just work, and you only live once!

> This pattern of being addicted to work will cause suffering in every area of your life because you are neglecting important aspects of your life, including your emotional development.

How many hours in the day are you working or thinking about work?

No. 7   A pattern of perfectionism and/or its bedfellow, procrastination

Are you a perfectionist? Are you a procrastinator?

We may expect perfection from ourselves and others, and believe that others expect perfection from us. We can also have a strong fear of failure or even fear success. Our self-worth is bound up in what we achieve, although what we achieve is never enough.

The strong fear of failure or success can often cause us to avoid doing things; or overdo them; or not finish them; or spend far too long doing them – all because we fear being judged not good enough, not perfect enough – a failure, even.

We may worry unduly, feel powerless and so end up doing nothing at all because we are afraid of failure. If we achieve perfection, we can then fear not being able to repeat this perfection and so avoid doing other things.

It is okay just to do your best. Who said that you had to be perfect? Nobody else is. You don't need to attribute so much importance to others' perception of you. You have to accept that good really is good enough – that good is perfect enough.

> This pattern can be a destructive force in your life, eroding your confidence and self-esteem.

No. 8   A pattern of over-readiness to please people and be over-responsible

Are you too ready to please others and take excessive responsibility?

We may take undue responsibility for others and their problems and respond to unreasonable demands, time and time again. We may constantly work too hard to please others or to gain acceptance from them. We may believe that others will like us better the more we carry for them – yet the more we carry, the more they seem to want us to carry. We may neglect our own needs in favour of others' and exhaust ourselves.

It's good to be able to give and take in life but it is of prime importance to take care of our own needs first.

> This pattern can leave us feeling unappreciated, resentful, taken advantage of, and a martyr.
>
> It can also hinder others from taking responsibility for themselves.

Are you able to say no and feel okay about it?

No. 9 A pattern of exaggerating the negative and minimising the positive

Do you exaggerate the negative and minimise the positive in your life?

We can exaggerate the frequency, intensity or importance of negative happenings in our life such as making a mistake, not getting the job we applied for, a simple confrontation or constructive criticism. We can also exaggerate someone else's achievements and minimise our own. We can compare ourselves unfavourably to others.

We can minimise the positives in our life or fail to recognise them – our own honourable qualities, abilities and achievements.

This pattern will crush our confidence and self-esteem.

Holding onto old unhelpful patterns of thinking that frequently stress and upset us is like sleeping on a hard lumpy mattress – not a good bedfellow!

When we exchange our cognitive distortions for more rational ways of thinking, our emotional reactions to situations become more hopeful.

We begin to feel a lot better in many areas of our life.

Did you read them all and think you had them all?

If you have identified a pattern or patterns in yourself, that's great. Move on to Resource 2.

Resource 2
Change Your Cognitive Distortions

The power of directed metaphorical stories

We will help you target each cognitive distortion using enjoyable, lighthearted, directed and metaphorical stories to change and update them.

Imprinting new desired patterns using directed metaphorical stories is one of the most effective ways to change, refine or update existing unhelpful patterns in the brain.

It is also the most effective way to create healthier patterns which we can build on.

Directed metaphorical stories have the built-in capacity to deliver multiple layers of complex, encoded messages and information. These stories appeal to the subconscious creative mind where all our patterns are stored. Our subconscious mind, with its pattern-recognition and matching ability, can use this information to reshape, change, update or delete specific targeted, unhelpful views and patterns.

Changing your cognitive distortions

All metaphorical stories that correspond to the cognitive distortions are in Resource 3.

● Your selected metaphorical story offers a new blueprint to your creative unconscious mind as a replacement for the old cognitive distortion.

- You will be able to see your pattern more clearly after reading the metaphorical story.
- You will be able to see where and how it impacts on your life.
- Only work with one cognitive distortion at a time until you change it.
- Relax – do your relaxing breathing first.

Exercise 1

Select and read the appropriate metaphorical story in **Resource 3** that corresponds to the specific cognitive distortion you have chosen to work on. For example:

If you choose cognitive distortion no. 2 then read the metaphorical story no. 2 (Quails & Snake) in **Resource 3**.

Now that you have read your relevant metaphorical story and you are able to see your cognitive distortion more clearly, go to Exercise 2.

Exercise 2

a Look at how your cognitive distortion affects you emotionally and how it affects your reactions and behaviour.
b In which kind of situations does the pattern mostly occur?
c How does your self talk reflect your identified pattern?
d How do you think it affects others involved?

Exercise 3

Confront and challenge your cognitive distortion

Cognitive distortions do not stand up to rational scrutiny because they are not rational.

a How do I know if this view is true? Is it based on fact?
b How is this view benefiting me now – my emotions, my health, my relationships, my happiness?
c How will it affect me in the future if I hold onto it?
d What are the negative consequences of holding onto this view?

Cognitive behavioural therapy (CBT) – become your own detective!

> You can tackle your own irrational thinking and behaviour in specific situations that distress you using the following cognitive behavioural therapy (CBT) format.

Once you see the negative consequences of your distorted view, you will be able to loosen its grip on you further and ultimately challenge and change it.

Whenever you find yourself getting upset, stressed, anxious or angry in a situation that wouldn't bother most people, ask yourself, **'how am I viewing the situation?'**

Example of a problematic situation caused by the cognitive distortion 'exaggerating the negative and minimising the positive'

a **You need to recognise what triggered your irrational thought pattern:**
Someone commented on your report at a meeting, saying it was too long-winded and detailed.

b **You need to be aware of your thoughts about the event:**
'I got it wrong. My report was crap. They will think I don't know what I am talking about and they will laugh at me behind my back. No one will say it to my face.'

c **You need to recognise the emotional consequences of thinking this way:**
Are you feeling anxious, upset or humiliated? Has your confidence taken a knock?

d **You need to recognise the behavioural consequences of thinking and feeling this way:**
'I am not going to go for a drink on the way home – I can't face my colleagues.'

Example of a better outcome to the problematic situation

Firstly, adopt a balanced, more realistic view of the situation.

a **Review the trigger:**
Someone commented on your report at a meeting, saying that it was too long-winded and detailed.

b **Change your view regarding the event – remind yourself of the truth:**
'No one disagreed about the content of my report. The reality was that people agreed with the points I made and had good discussions about them.'
Another truth:
'Only one person said that my report was too detailed and long-winded.'

c **Emotional consequences as a result of your realistic view:**
Feeling positive but a little disappointed.
Feeling good that people found that my report was very helpful and informative.

d **Your behavioural consequences now:**
'I can recognise my mistake and learn how to make my reports more concise.'
'I can go for a friendly drink with my colleagues on the way home and enjoy being with them.'

Final step to maintaining a healthy view

Be more aware of your unhelpful thought patterns and reactions, see them for what they are and challenge them.

If you have more than one cognitive distortion, choose the next one to work on and follow the same format as before.

Practise – the more you challenge them, the weaker they become until they finally change.

Resource 3
Metaphorical Stories Targeting Cognitive Distortions

Metaphorical stories to target specific cognitive distortions

By working on an image that reflects an irrational thinking pattern (cognitive distortion) and changing it into a more positive image, we automatically change the unhelpful thoughts, emotions and sensations that go along with it.

Now, sit down, put your feet up, relax and read the appropriate metaphorical story that corresponds to your specific chosen cognitive distortion.

No. 1   A pattern of black and white thinking – you view many things as either black or white

The Two Tin Soldiers

Tin Tom and Tin John were two brave tin soldiers, who had fought many a battle. One day, they decided to visit 'The Forest of Mystery and Beauty'.

They set off early in the misty dawn and chatted excitedly as they marched along the grassy forest path.

Tin Tom left his heavy armour behind him and carried only his silver sword. Tin John came fully-armoured and wearing his special tin glasses. These special glasses were made entirely of tin, even the lenses. He had made one tiny hole in the centre of each lens to see through.

As they marched along the forest path, the air was alive with the singing of red, blue, yellow, orange and green exotic birds. Insects flitted among the fresh green leaves of the trees and the brilliantly-coloured flowers. Tin Tom watched the beautiful birds and insects, feeling awe and wonderment.

Tin John, wearing his tin glasses, only saw the occasional bird that came within his direct line of pinhole vision. He became annoyed at his friend Tin Tom for pointing out different birds, insects and butterflies and the dappled sunlight that danced among the trees.

It was still early when the two tin soldiers came to the end of the path that led out of the forest. Tin Tom suggested that they explore other paths through the forest.

Tin John objected, saying that he had seen everything worth seeing in the forest and he was going back. Tin John, his tin armour clattering, marched back alone to his familiar camp — still wearing his tin glasses.

Alone, Tin Tom took the 'mystery path' in the forest and found it to be full of beauty and wonder. He stood to watch small birds feeding on mossy banks, which were bedecked with the most magnificent array of iridescent wild flowers. The exquisite scent in the air made his tin head buzz with sheer delight. He bathed in hot springs that dotted this landscape. He sat on a great white rock and felt the gentle heat of the sun and warm breeze soothe and caress his tin body. Small animals and butterflies came to welcome him as he sat on his rock. He ate some delicious fruit that grew in abundance along the bank of a sparkling clear stream.

It was late evening when Tin Tom came back to the camp feeling invigorated and full of wonder. He sat down beside his friend, Tin John, and told of his wonderful and exciting experiences. Tin John felt cheated by none other than himself and became distressed. He fell silent and, after some time, he began to cry – great loud sobs that echoed around the camp. Tin Tom sat beside him and didn't know what to say to console him; he reached out and just held his small tin hand.

After a while, Tin John stopped crying and spoke these words to his friend: 'Tin Tom, will you come to visit The Forest of Mystery and Beauty with me tomorrow? I missed so much beauty and wonder. His voice sounded croaky and shaky.

'Of course, I will,' said Tin Tom, all excited. 'There is so much beauty and wonder to see.'

When the two brave soldiers set out the following morning, there were no tin glasses with pinholes on Tim John. Both tin soldiers carried only their silver swords, which gleamed by their sides.

No. 2   A pattern of catastrophic thinking – a tendency to assume the worst

Quails & Snake

While a flock of Quails was engrossed in eating the juicy, purple-red berries that lay in abundance under the mulberry tree, Snake, who lived in a hole in the tree trunk, secretly watched them. Snake saw how happy the Quails were, hopping around joyfully and playfully while feasting on the mulberries.

It made Snake cross that the Quails were so happy. He himself was feeling bored and grumpy and wanted a bit of entertainment. He decided to terrify the Quails for his own amusement and pleasure. 'Stupid-looking birds,' he muttered to himself. 'I will teach you how to tremble before me; I will steal the happiness out of your hearts.' He slithered his scaly head and half his body out of his hole, startling the Quails.

In a voice that was filled with menace and foreboding, he announced, 'You have to stay here and grow fat; you are going to be my dinner. I cannot eat you now, you are too thin and scrawny, grow fat, grow fat quickly,' he bellowed. 'I am getting hungrier and hungrier.'

While he spoke, the Quails saw that his head puffed up dangerously and his flicking tongue darted about fiercely. His nostrils widened as he sniffed the air. He opened his jaws wide, displaying four big dangerous-looking fangs, hissed loudly and cast a pall of fear over the Quails. He then slithered silently and deliberately back into his hole and went to sleep.

The Quails trembled and became overwhelmed with fear. They were frantic and cried out to each other, 'Oh, oh, oh, Snake is going to get us, Snake is going to get us. We are doomed, we are doomed; we had better eat quickly, Snake is going to kill us, he ordered us to eat quickly and grow fat for him, oh, oh, Snake is going to kill us and eat us.'

The beautiful mulberries that had enchanted the Quails moments before became a nightmare to them. Frantically, the Quails started to eat the mulberries. Their fear intensified with each berry they ate. Many of them got bad diarrhoea from the fear. Some of them became so ill with the fear that they could not eat at all. Some of them jumped around, not knowing which mulberries to eat. Some of them got sick and vomited the mulberries. As the days passed, they became more frantic and fearful. All grew thinner and thinner.

Snake watched from his hole in the tree, pleased with the power he had over the Quails. He had always envied their ability to fly. He cackled with laughter and puffed himself up with pride. He laughed so much that his old head wobbled uncontrollably up and down. He hadn't known it would go so well.

One dark night, when fear among the Quails was so unbearable that they stood paralysed and helpless and unable even to pick at a single mulberry, the spirit of one tiny Quail woke up from its slumber and whispered urgently to the terrorised Quails.

'You are all able to escape, you have the gift of flight – fly – fly. You are still able to fly – Snake is tricking you. He can't fly – Snake can't fly.' No sooner had the words been spoken than the flock of Quails, flapping their wings, took to the air.

They did not stop until they landed on the side of their own familiar mountain. Although exhausted, their hearts were filled with joy because they were free from the false power Snake had over them. They vowed never to be tricked like that again.

No. 3   A pattern of over-sensitivity and jumping to wrong conclusions

Crow & Blackbird

Crow Matilda was feeling very happy one morning. It was bright and sunny and she felt the stirrings of an egg inside her belly. She spotted a blackbird trying to carry a clump of springy yellow moss in his beak to a nearby green leafy bush, where he was building a nest. The clump of moss was too big for the blackbird's beak and he dropped it in mid-flight. The blackbird took a quick sharp turn and flew down to try to pick it up again. Crow Matilda flew down and landed beside the blackbird.

'Noble effort,' said Matilda to the blackbird. She was very impressed with the blackbird for having found such springy yellow moss because it was very hard to come by. In her excitement about the lovely golden moss, she let out great peals of laughter and danced about. The blackbird froze on the spot and felt highly insulted, believing that the crow was poking fun at him.

'I only came to help you carry your fine moss,' said Matilda, who felt warmly towards this new friend.

The blackbird took even greater offence. 'Now ugly face crow with the crap voice thinks I am incapable of carrying my own moss,' he thought to himself. Angry and upset, the blackbird flew away, leaving the soft golden moss scattered on the ground.

'Oh!' Matilda sighed, 'I wish he would have let me carry the moss for him. I wanted to do a little act of kindness today for such a resourceful little blackbird. That way, he might have let me see how to make that soft, cosy, little nest he is building. I would like to learn how to weave soft moss for my family's nest, instead of the hard old twigs that we crows use.'

Later that day, the blackbird saw Matilda crow struggling to place a little bit of green moss among her stick nest. He saw the wind quickly whip the moss away and heard Matilda crow crying. He flew over to help her and showed her how to make a cosy mossy nest for her precious family. The blackbird and Matilda crow are now best friends.

No. 4 A pattern of guilt and self-blame
No. 5 A pattern of blaming others and avoiding responsibility

The Broken Eggs

The 10-year-old twins, Lolita and Monica, were sent to the shop to buy eggs for their mother's café. Lolita took a straw basket to carry the eggs in, rather than the strong plastic egg carrier her mother told her to take. Lolita hated the egg carrier – it wasn't cool. Monica tried to persuade her sister that the egg carrier was best but Lolita would have none of it and grabbed the straw basket.

They bought the eggs in the shop and both girls took a handle of the basket and set off for home.

Not far down the road, they spotted a blackberry bush laden with ripe juicy blackberries. They parked the basket on the ground and began to pick and eat the lovely blackberries. Lolita forgot the basket beside her feet and stepped into it, breaking many of the eggs.

'It is your stupid fault that the eggs are broken,' shouted Lolita at Monica. 'You wanted to pick the blackberries and that's why the eggs are broken now. If you hadn't wanted to pick the blackberries, I would never have stopped to pick them and I would not have put my foot in the basket and broken the eggs.'

'I know, I know,' said Monica, sobbing. 'It is all my fault—I'm to blame—I so wanted to pick the berries. I'm sorry.'

All evening, Monica felt guilty and blamed herself for the eggs that Lolita had broken by putting her foot into the basket. Full of remorse and guilt, she hid away in her room. Lolita played with her favourite games and had a good time.

Later that evening, Kiad, Monica's and Lolita's younger brother, came into Monica's room to see why she was hiding with the door closed. Monica was still very upset and told the whole story about the broken eggs to Kiad. She said that it was all her fault and now Mum was upset and angry with her.

Kiad threw his head back and laughed and laughed. 'You didn't break the eggs, Monica, you are crazy, what is wrong with you? It was the cunning Lolita who broke the eggs and as always, she tricked you into carrying the yoke. Ha, ha, ha.'

Soon Monica began to laugh, too, and they chased each other playfully around the house, singing, 'The yoke, the yoke has been passed around – I won't carry it – carry it – it can stay on the ground.'

Lolita heard them singing and came in to listen. 'What is the yoke?' she asked.

Monica replied, 'The yokes you put your foot in and then blamed me for – the same yokes you chose to put in the basket rather than the egg carrier.'

'You're right,' said Lolita. 'I thought I had got away with it again.'

She then began to sing, 'The yokes, the yokes have been passed around – I jumped in them and splashed them around!'

No. 6 A pattern of being addicted to work

The Hamster Clan

A group of hamsters lived in a large wooden hamster house in a beautiful meadow.

Their wooden house was very comfortable indeed and lined with the choicest soft hay and moss. They had several good exercise wheels in their house which they would use whenever the mood took them. The hamsters liked keeping strong, fit and agile so that they could jump and frolic in their beautiful meadow and the surrounding green rolling hills.

One hamster called Ludd wanted to prove that he could make the best ever hamster wheel. He said to himself, 'I shall make a wheel that will be a monument to myself. The wheel I shall fashion will make me a super hamster hero among the hamsters in the land. All the hamsters will be in awe of such a wonder – they will honour me. I know I can make a bigger and better wheel than any hamster, living or dead.' And so he set to work on his plans.

He called a meeting and told all the other hamsters in great detail about his plans. After repeatedly hearing about Ludd's plans, any future mention of them would send the hamsters scampering and frolicking into the meadow. Their indifference regarding this great wheel disappointed and perplexed Ludd.

With great gusto, Ludd began to build his great wheel. He worked on it night and day; he dreamt about it; and he talked non-stop about it – even though no one really listened. He hardly slept – he never went to the meadow any more, and neither did he play or frolic. He forgot to make new babies and couldn't remember what his children looked like.

He felt great making his wheel – excited, exhilarated. Frequently, he woke some of the hamsters from their slumber to help. After a short burst of energy the hamsters would run away down the meadow out of sight. He was dismayed by their lack of interest in his great wheel.

Finally, the wheel was complete and it was a good specimen indeed – Ludd himself was elated. None of the other hamsters honoured or praised Ludd for building the great wheel as they were too busy playing. Ludd was disappointed. He wanted every hamster to sing his praises.

He got up on his great wheel and round and round he went at high speed.

The other hamsters watched him in alarm – he was going too fast on his machine and wouldn't stop. The sweat was dripping off him, his body was getting thinner and weaker, he was puffing and panting, and his heart was crashing frantically against his rib cage. His old hamster friends watched him in dismay. In vain they begged him to stop and get off the wheel — he just shook his head and kept going.

One bright morning, without any warning, Ludd jumped off the wheel and staggered into the meadow. The morning dew sparkled like diamonds on the fresh meadow grass and flowers. He sat down and ate a bit of grass and a bright yellow daisy. They tasted so sweet and wonderful. He sniffed the fresh morning breeze and felt it lovingly dry his old sweaty wet coat. He lay on his back and looked up at the clear blue sky and heard the early morning skylarks singing in the new day.

He felt a lightness and a joy spring up in his little hamster heart – a joy he hadn't felt for a long time.

Such joy made him cry. His fellow hamsters were happy to have Ludd back as one of the gang. He grew stronger and healthier and never bothered any more with his super wheel.

No. 7   A pattern of perfectionism and/or it's bedfellow, procrastination

Magic Rain Clouds

The great King of the 'Small White Fluffy Clouds' blew his golden trumpet to call a group of them together to do a special, important task. The clouds gathered round the great King in readiness to do his bidding.

'I want you all to glide quickly across the sky and find the great water ocean in the land of plenty.'

'There, take in as much water as you can and then speed to the parched land of the Red people, where they are planting their crops, and drop your water. Without your water, the crops will wither and die in the burning sun and the people will starve.'

In haste, and calling on the power of the mighty winds, the clouds sped quickly across the sky to the great water ocean. However, one small white fluffy cloud called Monock did not move because he had decided to expand into a bigger shape to take in more water. So he waited and waited and waited. He didn't know when he had expanded enough so he waited and waited some more.

The other small white fluffy clouds, full-bellied with water, sped off, propelled by the wind, to the parched land of the Red people. They saw the parched earth below them and the Red people sitting, praying to the rain gods to come and water their newly-planted seeds before they died.

With great joy, the full-bellied white fluffy clouds rained down on the newly-planted seeds. They saw the Red people bow down in gratitude.

Without the help of the wind and his friends, Monock now thought it was time to go to the ocean. Without the wind, it was a struggle to get there.

When his belly was full of water, he went in search of the parched land of the Red people. It took him so long without the wind and his friends that, when he finally got there, his fellow clouds were already there with their third load of water.

Below, in the land of the Red people, the planted seeds had put forth strong green shoots. Just one more rainfall would bring them to harvest. All the other clouds happily rained down their collected water on the growing shoots again. Monock began to look for the perfect place among the growing shoots to empty his belly full of rain. He looked and looked but couldn't find the right spot, so he held on to his black belly full of water, which was very heavy indeed.

The other clouds gathered around him and told him that they were confused and bewildered by his antics. After a few moments of brooding silence, Monock opened his belly and heavy sheets of rain poured down onto the land.

His valuable water was taken in by the crops and they produced a good harvest that provided enough food for the Red people.

Monock felt light and a sense of happy freedom grew in his little cloud heart.

Over the years, Monock, together with his cloud friends, could be seen drifting and speeding across the skies to wherever they were needed.

No. 8   A pattern of over-readiness to please people and be over-responsible

The Ostriches

It had been a long, scorching hot summer in this arid land and the rivers had dried up to a trickle. Only one lake managed to retain some water and even this was reduced to a mere water-hole. A vicious crocodile kept guard over this water-hole and devoured many of the parched, terrified animals that were forced out of necessity to take the deadly risk of quenching their burning thirst there every night.

One night, a flock of Ostriches waited their chance at the water-hole. A female Ostrich named Ezzie took the risk of going first to the water's edge to give her fellow Ostriches a better chance of survival. That night, they all drank and managed to escape without harm. Ezzie was acclaimed for her generous spirit in going first to the water's edge. The next week, they did the same thing, Ezzie going first to make it easier for the others. But one night, just as they bent their heads down to drink, a loud voice boomed out from the deep water.

'I won't eat any of you Ostriches if each of you gives me one of your feathers every night. There are fifteen of you and I will have fifteen feathers every night. I want to make a feather bed for my lady love.'

The Ostriches trembled and quivered in fear but all lined up around the water-hole and the crocodile yanked one big feather out of their flesh. They winced and cringed in pain as their feathers were ripped from them.

The next morning, the Ostriches sat together, complaining about their pain and worrying about having to give a feather every night.

'I will go on my own,' said Ezzie.

'But Vicious Jaws crocodile needs fifteen feathers and you can only give one,' replied one of the female Ostriches.

'Don't worry,' Ezzie said, 'I shall give him fifteen of my own feathers tonight, one for each of you.'

They all voiced their gratitude to her.

'You are the very best,' they said. 'Thank you so much.' They gave her lots of pecks and kisses.

'It's nothing,' she said. 'What are a few feathers?'

Each night, Ezzie allowed Vicious Jaws to pluck fifteen feathers while the rest of the Ostriches drank safely from the water-hole. Ezzie's Ostrich friends got so used to her sacrificing herself on their behalf that they even forgot to thank her at times. Their ungratefulness made Ezzie very sad and angry but she never complained about it. On the nights when they remembered to show their gratitude she was very happy indeed.

One night, when Ezzie was too ill to have all fifteen of her feathers plucked, the other Ostriches expressed their disappointment in her. How could she not sacrifice herself for them on this occasion?

Ezzie vowed to try harder next time even though her flesh was torn and bleeding. Indeed, she did try harder and managed to continue giving her feathers so that they could be spared.

When Vicious Jaws the crocodile had enough feathers to build his nest, he told Ezzie that she didn't have to give any more feathers. Ezzie's heart sank when she heard the news but she couldn't figure out why such a sinking feeling came over her. Feather-plucking was a painful business and she didn't have many more feathers to give. Indeed, she was almost bald.

The other Ostriches kept out of her way from then on and were embarrassed by her quaint bald looks and blood-streaked flesh. It was the mating season among the Ostriches and not even one male Ostrich gave her a second glance. Ezzie's heart felt crushed and broken; she felt abandoned and became very ill. The hot sun scorched and ate into her bare skin leaving big red blisters that soon turned into running sores.

'After all I have given, no one cares about me now,' she sobbed desolately to herself. She tried to drag herself to the water-hole but was too weak and ill to reach it. Her throat was now parched and her eyes were bleeding from the burning sun.

A passing Warthog with large tusks and ever-watchful eyes spotted Ezzie lying helpless and alone on the burning scorched earth. He came over to sniff her; he was curious and had never seen such a featherless blistered Ostrich before.

He became very concerned. 'My dear, you are burning up and ill,' he said.

There was gentleness in his voice. 'Would you like me to take you back to my family so that you can grow strong again? We have only sparse hair and no feathers ourselves and know how to keep cool and well.'

Even in her weak state, Ezzie wanted to say she'd manage fine on her own. But, just for once, something different occurred and she said: 'Yes, I would like your help very much.' Without further ado the Warthog hoisted Ezzie on his back and hastened home with her.

In the cool dripping cavern of the Warthog's den, Ezzie was protected from the burning sun and given food and water. In the cool of the evenings, the young Warthogs taught her how to forage for food. She had never had it so good. There was such a variety of roots and seeds that she had never tasted before. She quickly grew healthy and strong and, soon beautiful shiny feathers began to grow on her. She played with the Warthogs and showed them all the games and dances she knew. The Warthogs were so proud and happy to be her friend and taught her lots of exciting new things in return.

When Ezzie was fully feathered, she went back to see the Ostrich clan. She walked among them with head held high. When a young, bossy male Ostrich tried to woo her, she just shook her head and said: 'You are not the one for me, dear.'

When some of the Ostriches asked her for some nesting feathers, she replied, 'Now you had better use your own, dear. Whatever gave you the idea that I would let you have feathers when you have got plenty of your own?'

Ezzie settled back in amongst her flock of Ostriches but she never forgot the lessons she had learned about unnecessarily pleasing others at her own expense. In the scarce, arid times, all the Ostriches shared equally the responsibility of going first to the water's edge.

Ezzie lived very happily with her fellow Ostriches to the end of her days. She never forgot her friends, the Warthogs, and went back to see them regularly.

No. 9   A pattern of exaggerating the negative and minimising the positive

The Crow Family

A pair of crows nested high up on a lovely tree close to an old farmer's barn in lush countryside. They were dedicated parents and hatched out two strong, healthy chicks, called Rudd and Doff.

For the past few weeks, the two young crows had been learning to fly in the green fields near the barn, closely supervised by their parents. Learning to fly was an exciting time for young Doff and Rudd and their joy and excitement spilled over into loud, gleeful squawks. They were almost as good at flying as their parents who were now proud and pleased at Rudd's and Doff's ability to fly so well.

One bright morning, as the two young crows had just taken off, Doff lightly brushed the barn wall with his wings. He landed on the ground with a squawk. It was evident that he hadn't really hurt himself because he got up quickly and hopped around playfully.

On seeing Doff's light brush with the wall, the parents were devastated and brought the two young crows back up into their nest in the tree for safety.

'You are not yet ready to learn how to fly,' Mother crow said in a shaky voice. Their father nodded in agreement. 'You will have another accident and kill yourself — we shall have to stay close to the nest and teach you first to hop safely on the nearby branches. After some weeks, you may be able to come down into the green field again but it may take a long time. We shall stay with you,' said mother Crow reassuringly. 'Rudd will have to stay here as well and learn how to fly, too.'

Doff and Rudd together began to squawk and shout: 'We can both fly – we have been flying in the green field and up into the tree for a few weeks now. This was just one small mishap.'

'That's the end of it,' said the parents, 'you are both staying here where you will be safe.'

Both young crows tried to tell their parents about all the flying abilities they already had and they pleaded with their parents to allow them down to fly in the green field. It was all to no avail – the parents refused.

Doff and Rudd were so upset and cross that they even tried to rip up their nest. A few pecks on the heads by their parents stopped them.

As evening fell, the parent crows went off to collect food for Doff and Rudd. As soon as the parent crows left the nest, Rudd and Doff escaped and flew across the fields together in the dancing evening sunlight. They spotted some pigeons feasting on sweet grain in a corn field and flew down to join them. Doff and Rudd never went home that night.

Next day, they flew back together to their lovely field and the old barn. Their worried parents were delighted to see them again and didn't know what to say to them.

'We are really good at flying,' said Doff.

'We are,' said Rudd, 'and our wings are growing stronger every day.'

'Soon we will be great flyers,' said Doff.

'We will be great flyers,' said Rudd.

Suddenly, both crow parents realised the truth – that Rudd and Doff had many flying abilities already and were growing stronger in flight every day. The following day, Doff and Rudd, together with their parents, found great joy in making a long flight to the magic faraway mountain.

Resource 4
How To Change Four 'Untrue' Core Beliefs And Feel Great

Targeting untrue core beliefs

We will again use directed imagery and metaphorical stories to target and change the **four major untrue core beliefs** that, for the most part, determine our self-esteem and our happiness.

> Your unconscious mind and your own imagination are your most powerful allies in helping you change any untrue core beliefs you may hold about yourself.

Targeting the imagery and metaphors that reflect *untrue core beliefs* in our unconscious mind and transforming them into more helpful images or metaphors will enable our unconscious mind to delete or update them. Our unconscious mind will soon adopt the *new true core beliefs* as new blueprints to follow. For example, if you have a deep-seated unconscious belief that you are not as valuable as others, this *untrue core belief* in your unconscious mind can be transformed into the *new true core belief* that you are in fact equally as valuable as others. Just by changing that *one belief* about yourself, so many things in your life will change for the better.

Our four major core beliefs that are the key to our happiness

> The four major core beliefs related to our self-esteem are the beliefs that form the basic assumptions we make about:
>
> a how lovable, equally valid and worthwhile we are
> b how much security we imagine we have
> c how much personal power we think we have
> d how capable we believe we are

(See Chapter 23 'Self-Esteem – Your Key To A Happier Life' and Chapter 24 'Our Unconscious Beliefs')

It's important to become aware of any untrue core beliefs you hold about yourself

- All of us hold some of these *untrue core beliefs*. Many of us hold more. Work on the ones that apply to your life and you will soon feel stronger.

- Once you recognise any *untrue core beliefs* you hold, you are halfway to changing them. You will be amazed at how much insight into them and motivation to change them you already possess.

- Weakening them and changing them is much easier than you imagine and we will show you how to do this in light-hearted, humorous and positive ways that really work well.

- You will be able to recognise these *untrue core beliefs* in your repeated negative thoughts and your repetitive negative *self talk* about yourself.

- You will also be able to recognise them if you frequently have strong unwarranted emotional reactions, such as anxiety, fear, anger, guilt or shame, to situations that wouldn't bother most people.

Only work on one *untrue core belief* at a time.

Be persistent in doing the exercise for changing each *untrue core belief* – repetition is key, as is talking kindly to yourself.

Every time you work on an *untrue core belief*, you will weaken its grip on you. Remember, it is your key to greater self-esteem and a happier, more fulfilling life.

It doesn't matter how long you have had an *untrue core belief* about yourself. You can still change it and re-discover more of the real you – your authentic, powerful self.

Please remember, if you have difficulty dealing with any aspect of your life and feel held back, it is courageous and brave to seek professional help. We would strongly advise this. We are all human, we all suffer and we all need help at times.

The following Resources 4a, 4b, 4c and 4d will enable you to recognise, eliminate and change any of the four major untrue core beliefs that you hold.

Resource 4a
Core Belief No. 1
Love Yourself More

Core Belief No. 1 **How lovable, equally valid and worthwhile do you feel?**

Check out these examples of repetitious thoughts and self talk that reflect an untrue core belief about how lovable, equally valid and worthwhile you are:

- No one **will ever** really love me; no one **has ever** really loved me; some people are nice to me because they feel sorry for me; I don't even love myself; I hate myself.
- Nothing good ever happens to me. What I need is not important.
- Other people are more deserving than me. People always reject me.
- Other people are much better than me. I feel crap about myself – ugly and undesirable.
- To feel worthwhile, I need to achieve well, otherwise people will not approve of me.
- If I please people and get everything right, they may accept me and like me better.
- I am flawed and damaged and I feel a fake. If people really knew me, they would not like me – I can't let people see who I am.
- To feel better, I always need to succeed at what I do. If I try and fail, people will think I am crap and stupid.
- I need to work harder than anyone else to prove myself.

Change your untrue core belief about how lovable, equally valid and worthwhile you are

Now you can learn to love yourself a bit more. Without this, we can put ourselves down, resort to harsh judgments, condemn ourselves, feel insecure and make unfavourable comparisons with others.

To compensate for our lack of self-regard, we can place too much importance on pleasing others, take on too much responsibility and put our own needs on hold.

Exercise I Love yourself more – give your unconscious mind a healthier perspective on your true value and worth

Sit down and make yourself comfortable and take a few relaxing breaths and breathe peace into your heart. Imagine that you are now in your own lovely peaceful haven (see page 25), sitting on your chair.

> Remind yourself that these negative feelings about your true value and worth are not based on truth but mostly on the conclusions you came to as a young child.

Ponder this now: we are **all** equally valuable human beings deserving of love and respect and a happy life. No one is superior to you, or better than you, unless they are deluded! Realise fully that no human being is perfect and you don't have to be. We are all unique and we do not need to compare ourselves unfavourably with others. We can learn to love ourselves and treat ourselves and others with compassion and kindness. Then our hearts will be much happier and our self-esteem will grow.

Read your metaphorical story now, slowly and peacefully and let your creative unconscious mind begin to do its great, transforming work.

The Three Dolls

Three dolls came to pay homage to the great Queen of the world and to receive her wisdom.

Two of the dolls were dressed in the finest silk. They wore red, green and golden robes. Sparkling diamonds hung round their necks on golden chains. The neat little shoes on their feet were bedecked with pearls.

The third doll was dressed in torn black rags, her hair was all matted, and her feet were bare and dirty. Her face was dirty, too, and streaked with tears.

The Queen asked the dolls to walk forward one by one and say their names.

The first doll walked towards the Queen with head held high and said, 'My name is Faith.' The Queen smiled and said, 'A very good name indeed.'

The second doll stepped forward with her head held high and said, 'My name is Hope.' The Queen smiled. 'It is a good name indeed,' said the Queen.

The third and last doll, with her tattered clothes and matted hair, stepped forward with head bowed.

'My name is Nobody,' she said.

The Queen did not speak, looked sad and closed her eyes for a few moments.

The Queen asked all the dolls to turn round slowly one by one.

Faith turned round first and the back of her dress was torn and in shreds, while the back of her hair was matted and dirty.

Hope turned round. The back of her dress was torn and in tatters, while her hair was dirty and matted.

Finally, Nobody turned round.

The back of her dress was a magnificent green and gold colour and made of pure silk and her hair was golden, clean, smooth and shining.

The other two dolls had never seen how beautiful Nobody was before – they gasped in amazement.

The Queen smiled at the dolls.

She took Nobody's little hands in hers and told her that, from now on, her name was 'Love'. The doll smiled happily and nodded her head.

'You are all truly great dolls – real dolls indeed,' said the Queen, 'perfect as you are.'

She gave each of the little dolls a wonderful gift of a very special mirror. This mirror allowed them to see all of themselves, back, front and sides.

They treasured their gifts forever. Their gifts gave each of them the power eventually to run and even fly high up in the sky.

After you have read the metaphorical story, take a few relaxing breaths and be at peace there in your safe haven for about five minutes. Then move on to Exercise 2.

Exercise 2   Eliminate your untrue core belief that makes you feel less lovable, less valuable and less worthy than others

Affirm to yourself: 'I now choose to eliminate my untrue core belief that I am less lovable, less valuable and less worthy than others.'

Familiarise yourself first with this exercise. Take a few relaxing, calming breaths and send love to your heart. Imagine that you are still in your quiet, calm, safe haven ......

- Imagine that in your garden you have a nice oak table and chair. On your table you have a bottle of deep blue ink, a gold pen and a sheet of cream parchment.
- You pick up the parchment and feel its cool crispness and velvety touch between your fingers. It smells fresh and new.
- You sit down on your chair and slowly and carefully write on your parchment:

'I now choose to eliminate my untrue core belief that I am less lovable, less valuable and less worthy than others.'

- You fold up the parchment carefully and put it into the black cardboard box that is there on the table close by.
- You hold the box in your hands and make your way carefully along a little path to the end of your garden. Here, a small, intense fire burns brightly in a steel drum.

- You dump your box into the heart of the bright glowing flames and watch as your box containing your old belief is quickly consumed and turned into white ash.
- You feel great relief and peace.
- You walk back to your chair in the garden and sit at your oak table.

Take a few relaxing breaths now and stay in your peaceful, safe haven, breathing and relaxing for a few moments. Then move on to the next exercise.

Exercise 3   Create your new true core belief: 'I am an equally lovable, valuable and worthy human being'

> Affirm to yourself your new true core belief: 'I now choose to believe that I am an equally lovable, valuable and worthy human being.'

Imagine that, on your table, is a silver dish containing seven big, bright, beautiful rainbow-coloured seeds called the **'Seeds of Self-Love and Self-Regard'**.

Attached to the dish is a white label with red writing on it that says, 'The true core belief that I am an equally lovable, valuable and worthy human being.'

They are the shiniest seeds you have ever seen and there is a warm glow coming from them – you can feel their warmth when you pick them up in your hand.

Take a few relaxing breaths again.

Now imagine ......
- You walk over to a patch of earth nearby that is prepared and ready for planting.
- With your finger you make holes about 2 cm deep in the fresh, brown, warm earth and pop a seed in each hole.

- You scoop some rich compost out of the bucket beside you and gently put it over each seed, patting the earth flat.
- You use the little watering-can that is close by to sprinkle water over the soil.
- Now, sit back and breathe peacefully in your chair in your safe haven and just enjoy being there for a short while.

Then imagine ......
- That you revisit your patch of earth where you planted your seeds and see the amazing, vibrant, pink flowers that have bloomed so quickly – smell their scent, touch their soft petals, observe their bright, vibrant, green stems and leaves – enjoy them!

When you are ready, count backwards from 10 to 1 and be fully in the present.

Spend a few quiet moments with yourself and determine to become your own best friend and to be kind and loving to yourself no matter what.

Talk kindly and positively to yourself and make this your daily practice.

Send love to your unique, beautiful heart.

Try to repeat these few exercises daily for a few weeks, or whenever you want to strengthen your self-love.

Resource 4b
Core Belief No. 2
Gain More Inner Security

Core Belief No. 2   How much inner security do you feel you have?

Check out these examples of repetitious thoughts and self talk that reflect an untrue core belief about how much inner security you have:

- I feel I have no control.
- Others can't be trusted – I have to watch my back all the time.
- I am a born worrier. I worry about everything – what others think of me, what they say, what I have said or done, and what I didn't say or didn't do.
- I can't cope with these types of situations – there is so much to worry about.
- If it's not one worry, it's another.
- I never feel at ease, I can't relax.
- Even in bed my head is full of worries – I worry all the time.
- I need constant reassurance from others.

Change your untrue core belief regarding your inner security

We all feel insecure at times. This is a common human trait, which only differs in degree between people.

Untrue core beliefs about your inner security can make you feel unduly anxious and worried about everyday situations. They can falsely make you feel that you have no control and so you may begin to rigidly control yourself, others or your environment. Ongoing insecurity can make many things in your life more difficult, such as making decisions, relationships, socialising, and doing something new. It can make you think negatively about yourself and about others, too.

A high degree of insecurity could make you mistrust life and the future. You might be perpetually wary of being picked on or hurt.

When we take the right action, despite our insecurity, to solve our problems and face challenging situations, we lessen our anxieties and strengthen our inner security.

Exercise 1   Give your unconscious mind a better perspective on your own inner security

Sit down and make yourself comfortable. Take a few relaxing breaths and breathe peace into your heart. Imagine that you are now in your own lovely peaceful haven (see page 25) sitting on your chair.

Remind yourself that all the negative thoughts and self talk that feed your insecurities are not always truths. They are thoughts mostly based on the conclusions of a young child.

Read your metaphorical story now, slowly and peacefully and let your creative unconscious mind begin to do its great, transforming work.

The Big Wheel

One day, a woman called Eliza Grey, found herself high up and alone on a very big Ferris wheel in a fairground. She didn't even know how she got there. No other human being or even an animal was in sight. The big wheel began speeding round and round at a rapid pace and made frightening metallic clattering noises as it was spinning.

It began to spin even faster and faster. Eliza Grey hung on for dear life. Her arm muscles were shaking and her knuckles were white from her tight grip on the iron bar in front of her.

The horrible rotten smell of a rubbish dump nearby made her feel nauseated. Her heart was pounding in her chest and cold sweat trickled down her face and into her eyes. The thought of being stuck there forever terrified her.

In fear and desperation, she released one hand from the bar that she was gripping so tightly, and with her free hand, she felt around the edge of her seat. Her groping hand found a big lever there. Struggling and pulling, she managed to flip the lever over to the opposite direction.

The big wheel made loud groaning noises and began to slow down – going slower and slower and slower. Finally it stopped, bringing a flood of relief that literally swept through Eliza Grey's body and made her feel all floppy.

She jumped off the big wheel and landed safely on the ground. With shaking legs and trembling body, she began to walk away from the wheel and away from the rubbish dump. She soon found herself approaching a beautiful calm seafront.

She noticed some children and their parents playing in the rock pools further along the shore. Here, the sun shone brightly and the sky was bright blue above; the sea was calm and sparkled in the sunlight that danced on the water. She breathed the beautiful sea air into her lungs, sat down on the golden warm sand, looked towards the sea and felt very peaceful indeed.

After you have read the metaphorical story, take a few relaxing breaths and be at peace there in your safe haven for about five minutes. Then move on to Exercise 2.

Exercise 2   Eliminate your untrue core belief that makes you feel unduly insecure

Affirm to yourself: 'I now choose to eliminate my untrue core belief that feeds my insecurity.'

Familiarise yourself first with this exercise. Take a few relaxing, calming breaths and send love to your heart. Imagine that you are still in your quiet, calm, safe haven .....

- Imagine that in your garden you have a nice oak table and chair. On your table you have a bottle of deep blue ink, a gold pen and a sheet of cream parchment.
- You pick up the parchment and feel its cool crispness and velvety touch between your fingers. It smells fresh and new.
- You sit down on your chair and slowly and carefully write on your parchment:

  'I now choose to eliminate my untrue core belief that feeds my insecurity.'

- You fold up the parchment carefully and put it in the black cardboard box that is there on the table close by.
- You hold the box in your hands and make your way carefully along a little path to the end of your garden where a small intense fire burns brightly in a steel drum.
- You dump your box into the heart of the bright glowing flames and watch as your box containing your old belief is quickly consumed and turned into white ash.
- You feel great relief and peace.
- You walk back to your chair in the garden and sit at your oak table.

Take a few relaxing breaths now and stay in your peaceful, safe haven, breathing and relaxing for a few moments. Then move on to the next exercise.

Exercise 3 Create your new true core belief: 'I can be more secure'

Affirm to yourself your new true core belief:'I now choose to increase my feelings of inner security.'

Imagine that, on your table, is a dish containing big, bright, beautiful blue seeds called the '**Seeds of Inner Security**'.

Attached to the dish is a big white label with red print on it that says, 'The true core belief that I can increase my feeling of inner security'.

They are the shiniest seeds you have ever seen and there is a warm, deep-blue glow coming from them – you can feel the warmth when you pick them up.

Take a few relaxing breaths again.

Now imagine ......
- You walk over to a patch of earth not far from you that is prepared and ready for planting.
- With your finger you make holes about 2 cm deep in the fresh, brown, warm earth and pop a seed in each hole.
- You scoop some rich compost out of the bucket beside you and gently put it over each seed, patting the earth flat.
- You use the little watering-can that is close by to sprinkle water over the soil.
- Now, sit back and breathe peacefully in your chair in your safe haven and just enjoy being there for a short while.

Then imagine ......
- That you revisit your patch of earth where you have planted your seeds and see the amazing vibrant blue flowers that have bloomed so quickly – smell their scent, touch their soft petals, observe their bright, vibrant, green stems and leaves – enjoy them!

When you are ready, count backwards from 10 to 1 and be fully in the present.

Spend a few quiet moments realising that you can build up your inner security by learning how to control your stress, solving your problems, taking chances in life, trying new things and not taking it too seriously if things don't go to plan.

Talk kindly and positively to yourself and make this your daily practice.

Send love to your unique, beautiful heart.

Try to repeat these few exercises daily for a few weeks, or whenever you want to strengthen your feelings of inner security.

Resource 4c
Core Belief No. 3
Get Your Real Power Back

Core Belief No. 3   How much personal power do you feel you have?

Check out these examples of repetitious thoughts and self talk that reflect an untrue core belief regarding your personal power:

- I am powerless – my hands are tied. There is nothing at all I can do now.
- There is nothing I can change, I have to stick with it.
- There is no hope, things will never get better – I am just fooling myself, I always end up the loser no matter how hard I try.
- Everyone else seems to get what they want.
- I am a victim of circumstances, people always pick on me, and I get the worst deals.
- If I stand up for myself, he/she/they will take it out on me so there is no point in saying anything.
- Nothing turns out right for me.
- People always take from me and give nothing back.
- People always put upon me.
- I have to do others' work as well as my own.
- I never have time for myself.
- People always take advantage of me.
- Nobody pays any heed to what I want.

Change your untrue core belief regarding your personal power

You can take back more of your own personal power now. You may well have given it to others, allowing them to dominate you, undermine or take advantage of you. You may have difficulty standing up for yourself or saying no.

An untrue belief regarding your personal power may make you feel that you have no control or power in many situations; make you operate below par; make you believe there isn't anything that you can do to change things. You will lose out on many opportunities and chances. However, you are a lot more powerful than you imagine.

Exercise 1   Give your unconscious mind a true view of your personal power

Sit down and make yourself comfortable. Take a few relaxing breaths and breathe peace into your heart. Imagine that you are now in your own lovely peaceful haven (see page 25) sitting on your chair.

Begin to realise that all the negative thoughts and self talk regarding your personal power are not truths but mostly based on the conclusions of a young child.

Read your metaphorical story now, slowly and peacefully and let your creative unconscious mind begin to do its great, transforming work.

The Tethered Eagle

Imagine that you are the owner of a beautiful golden eagle. His feathers are dark brown and he has light golden-brown plumage on his head and neck.

You keep him in your back garden, tethered to a wooden post with a cord tied round his feet. He stays on his perch all day and night and all winter, spring, summer and autumn. His wings that once knew the freedom of the skies, mountains and valleys, his great wings that once glided and sailed with the wind, are now drooping, unkempt and dishevelled.

You see him regularly pick at, and tear, his own flesh with his sharp yellow beak – he is covered in sores.

You never hear his call any more and you wonder if his voice has been silenced forever.

As you look into his sad eyes – eyes that are capable of seeing vast distances and faraway horizons – you feel overwhelmed with pity for this once magnificent rider of the sky.

It's a beautiful day and the eagle is so dejected that he doesn't even look up at the bright blue sky above him.

At times you notice that he flaps his wings and frantically tries to fly. The rope around his legs is strong and holds him back — the effort exhausts him. You touch his feathers and they feel sticky and rough. You watch him peck listlessly at the food you give him and scatter most of it onto the ground.

You cannot bear to watch the plight of this great bird any more. It fills your heart with great sadness and fear – 'fear' because you realise that you are his captor.

You feel scared to take hold of this great eagle in case he pecks you with his sharp beak or claws you with his hooked talons.

Despite your fears, you get a big pair of scissors, grab hold of the fluttering eagle and cut off the tethers holding him captive.

At first he can't believe that his legs are free and he is no longer tied to the post. He inspects his legs and moves them about, lifting them up and down as if dancing. He stretches his wings wide — the widest you have ever seen him stretch.

He lets out his mighty call and takes to the sky, going higher and higher. You stand to watch him playing freely on the air currents high up in the sky.

After you have read the metaphorical story, take a few relaxing breaths and be at peace there in your safe haven for at least five minutes. Then move on to Exercise 2.

Exercise 2   Eliminate your untrue core belief that makes you feel powerless so often

> Affirm to yourself: 'I now choose to eliminate my untrue core belief that I am powerless.'

Familiarise yourself first with this exercise. Take a few relaxing, calming breaths – send love to your heart. Imagine that you are still in your quiet, calm, safe haven …...

* Imagine that in your garden you have a nice oak table and chair. On your table you have a bottle of deep blue ink, a gold pen and a sheet of cream parchment.
* You pick up the parchment and feel its cool crispness and velvety touch between your fingers. It smells fresh and new.
* You sit down on your chair and slowly and carefully write on your parchment:

   'I now choose to eliminate my untrue core belief that I am powerless.'

* You fold up the parchment carefully and put it in the black cardboard box that is there on the table close by.
* You hold the box in your hands and make your way carefully along a little path to the end of your garden where a small intense fire burns brightly in a steel drum.
* You dump your box into the heart of the bright glowing flames and watch as your box containing your old belief is quickly consumed and turned into white ash.
* You feel great relief and peace.
* You walk back to your chair in the garden and sit at your oak table.

Take a few relaxing breaths now and stay in your peaceful, safe haven, breathing and relaxing for a few moments. Then move on to the next exercise.

Exercise 3   Create your new true core belief: 'I have strong personal power'

Affirm to yourself your new true core belief: 'I choose to believe that I have strong personal power.'

Imagine that, on your table, is a dish containing big, bright, beautiful red seeds called the '**Seeds of Personal Power**'.

Attached to the dish is a big white label with red print on it that says, 'The true core belief that I have strong personal power'.

They are the shiniest seeds you have ever seen and there is a powerful energy coming from them when you pick them up.

Take a few relaxing breaths again.

Now imagine ......
- You walk over to a patch of earth not far from you that is prepared and ready for planting.
- With your finger you make holes about 2 cm deep in the fresh, brown, warm earth and pop a seed in each hole.
- You scoop some rich compost out of the bucket beside you and gently put it over each seed, patting the earth flat.
- You use the little watering-can that is close by to sprinkle water over the soil.
- Now, sit back and breathe peacefully in your chair in your safe haven and just enjoy being there for a short while.

Then imagine ......

- That you revisit your patch of earth where you have planted your seeds and see the amazing vibrant red flowers that have bloomed so quickly – smell their scent, touch their soft petals, observe their bright vibrant green stems and leaves – enjoy them!

When you are ready, count backwards from 10 to 1 and be fully in the present.

- Spend a few quiet moments realising your personal power is increased when you take action despite your fears.

- Every time you stand up for yourself or for others; every time you try new things or take a chance in life; every time you tell the truth when it is easier to lie, you are using and increasing your personal power.

- When you take full responsibility for your own health and happiness, you are exerting your personal power and increasing it.

- Talk kindly and positively to yourself and make this your daily practice.

- Send love to your unique, beautiful heart.

- Try to repeat these few exercises daily for a few weeks, or whenever you want to strenghten your personal power.

Resource 4d
Core Belief No. 4 Realise How Capable You Are

Core Belief No. 4   How capable do you feel you are?

Check out these examples of repetitious thoughts and self talk that reflect an untrue core belief about your capability:

- I am a failure.
- Better not to do it than to fail at it.
- I can't do anything right. I mess up everything.
- What is the point of even trying?
- It's too hard to learn something new.
- I have never been that good at anything.
- I am not as clever as others.
- I just get by and pretend.
- I can't do that. I wouldn't be good at it.
- It's too much of an effort. I would only fail at it anyhow.
- There is not much point in trying – I give up.
- It's a waste of time applying for that job as I won't get it anyway.
- I am stuck with this job. There is nothing else I am able to do.

Change your untrue core belief regarding your capability

With this pattern you may avoid new challenges or anything difficult. A setback may make you quickly lose confidence and give up trying. Remember that we learn best through trial and error and renewed, determined effort. To realise this you only have to watch a small child learning to walk.

Taking action, even though you might feel anxious about learning and trying out new things, is great for developing your capability.

Even as adults, we often mistakenly rate our capability according to how well we have done academically or what we have acquired materially so far, but these are not the only measures of success. We are all unique and there are many different ways in which we can develop our capabilities, talents, resources and positive qualities.

Exercise 1   Give your unconscious mind a healthier perspective on your true capability

Sit down and make yourself comfortable. Take a few relaxing breaths and breathe peace into your heart. Imagine that you are now in your own lovely peaceful haven (see page 25) sitting on your chair.

> Begin to realise that all the negative thoughts and self talk that feed your repetitive feelings of being incapable are not truths but are mostly based on the conclusions of a young child.
>
> You are far more capable and resourceful than you ever imagined and you can be courageous and a hero when you need to be.
>
> You have vast untapped capabilities and resources inside you.

Read your metaphorical story now, slowly and peacefully and let you creative unconscious mind begin to do its great, transforming work.

Going Through The Jungle

Imagine that you find yourself standing in front of a jungle. The river behind you is a raging torrent from all the rain; there is no way back.

Heavy rain is beating down on you – you are soaking wet. You have no map to tell you how far the jungle stretches or which direction will lead you out. You feel lost and really afraid. All you are carrying with you is a sharp-bladed, long-handled cutlass.

You decide to go forward. You start frantically slashing briars, twisted vines, spiky shrubs and plants to make a path for yourself. It is hard going, you are covered in sweat and your hands are getting hot and blistered as they are being prodded and scratched by the unfriendly thorns and spiky bushes in the thick undergrowth. The powerful acrid smells from the slashed shrubs and plants are overwhelming — the humidity is unbearable. You feel short of air and take in big gulping breaths at times.

You feel weak and light-headed with hunger. To your relief, you spot a strawberry guava bush nearby, laden with dripping, wet, juicy fruit.

You grab a few handfuls of the berries. Their juicy tartness is welcome refreshment for your parched mouth. They satisfy your desperate hunger and give you strength and energy to keep slashing.

You hear the rustle of animals scurrying away, startled by the slashing sounds. You see a big yellow and black snake slithering away to hide in the dense undergrowth to your left.

Despite exhaustion and bites in a thousand places from blood-sucking insects, you keep going. By evening, to your great relief, you abruptly arrive at the edge of the jungle.

The rain has stopped and a bright warm sun is shining. You look up to a bright blue sky above.

You see a sturdy golden bridge nearby leading across the river. You walk across the bridge and come to a road. You hear the laughter and voices of children nearby. A short distance up the road, you come to a beautiful town with lots of street cafés where people are laughing and chatting and eating.

They welcome you and listen attentively to your story in amazement. A hotel owner lets you shower and people bring you comfortable clothes to wear. You eat heartily with them and are overjoyed.

After you have read the metaphorical story, take a few relaxing breaths and be at peace there in your safe haven for at least five minutes. Then move on to Exercise 2.

Exercise 2 Eliminate your untrue core belief that makes you feel less than capable

Affirm to yourself: 'I now choose to eliminate my untrue core belief that says I am not a very capable person.'

Familiarise yourself first with this exercise. Take a few relaxing, calming breaths and send love to your heart. Imagine that you are still in your quiet, calm, safe haven …...

- Imagine that in your garden you have a nice oak table and chair. On your table you have a bottle of deep blue ink, a gold pen and a sheet of cream parchment.
- You pick up the parchment and feel its cool crispness and velvety touch between your fingers. It smells fresh and new.
- You sit down on your chair and slowly and carefully write:

  'I choose to eliminate the untrue core belief that I am not a very capable person'

- You fold up the parchment carefully and put it in the black cardboard box that is there on the table close by.
- You hold the box in your hands and make your way carefully along a little path to the end of your garden where a small intense fire burns brightly in a steel drum.
- You dump your box into the heart of the bright glowing flames and watch as your box containing your old belief is quickly consumed and turned into white ash.
- You feel great relief and peace.
- You walk back to your chair in the garden and sit at your oak table.

Take a few relaxing breaths now and stay in your peaceful, safe haven, breathing and relaxing for a few moments. Then move on to the next exercise.

Exercise 3 Create your new true core belief: 'I am a capable person who can learn and grow'

> Affirm to yourself your new true core belief: 'I choose to believe that I am a capable person who can learn and grow.'

Imagine that, on your table, is a dish containing big, bright, beautiful golden-yellow seeds called the **'Seeds of Capability'**.

Attached to the dish is a big white label with red print on it that says, 'The true core belief that I am a capable person who can learn and grow'.

They are the shiniest seeds you have ever seen and there is a warm glow coming from them – you can feel the warmth when you pick them up.

Take a few relaxing breaths again.

Now imagine ......
- You walk over to a patch of earth not far from you that is prepared and ready for planting.
- With your finger you make holes about 2 cm deep in the fresh, brown, warm earth and pop a seed in each hole.
- You scoop some rich compost out of the bucket beside you and gently put it over each seed, patting the earth flat.
- You use the little watering-can that is close by to sprinkle water over the soil.
- Now, sit back and breathe peacefully in your chair in your safe haven and just enjoy being there for a short while.

Then imagine ......
- That you revisit your patch of earth where you have planted your seeds and see the amazing vibrant golden-yellow flowers that have bloomed so quickly – smell their scent, touch their soft petals, observe their bright vibrant green stems and leaves – enjoy them!

When you are ready, count backwards from 10 to 1 and be fully in the present.

- Spend a few quiet moments with yourself, determined to view any problem or undertaking as a challenge that will make you more courageous, efficient and strong.

- Take action to deal with these challenges and problems in the best possible way.

- Don't get put off by a few setbacks, we all have them – dust yourself down and keep going!

- Ask for help if you need it.

- Put determined effort into improving your skills and abilities – these will continue to evolve throughout life.

- Talk kindly and positively to yourself and make this your daily practice.

- Send love to your unique, beautiful heart.

- Try to repeat these few exercises daily for a few weeks, or whenever you want to strengthen your capability.

Resource 5
Meditation To Balance Your Busy Mind

Meditation – a powerful de-stressor

Meditation is a well-used and powerful de-stressor recognised world-wide. Meditation allows us to switch off our constant mind chatter and relax. When our mind is quiet we are able to experience inner peace and calm even in the midst of chaos.

Don't be put off by the word 'meditation'. It is not something mysterious and you do not need to follow any particular religion or creed to practise it. You can meditate anywhere, any time. It is very easy to learn and, with a little practice, you will be able to incorporate it into your daily life.

Meditation can ease your troubled mind

Meditation is a very powerful tool that will help you reduce overall stress levels and enable you to release troubling feelings of anxiety and worry. Meditation creates a state of restful alertness where the mind and body are in a state of calm and rest but you remain completely aware. The inner calm and feelings of well-being that meditation brings will help you feel more positive and enable you to gain a better perspective on stressful events.

Meditation will help your immune system

You are now aware that there is a strong link between our state of mind and our physical health. In giving you peace of mind and reducing stress levels, meditation helps you avoid many stress-related illnesses. Meditation will boost your immune system – your body's natural defence against disease. It will help your body repair itself and minimise further damage.

There are many forms of meditation but all strive to achieve the same thing – a quiet, calm mind.

Meditation exercises

Any one of the following three simple meditations, even if practised for only five minutes a day, can have a profound effect on reducing your immediate stress as well as your long-term worries. With practice, you will be able to extend these five minutes to a longer period of time.

You may prefer to create or use any of your own meditations.

Meditation I   Focus on your breathing

- Sit comfortably in a quiet place, feet planted on the floor and eyes closed.
- Take some relaxing breaths first for a few moments. Breathe in to a count of 5 and breathe out slowly to a count of 9, and then begin to breathe normally.
- Now just observe your breathing – notice the in and out flow of your breath.
- Don't try to change anything – just observe. Nothing is right or wrong – there is nothing to do or change – just observe the in flow and the out flow of your breath.
- If your mind wanders, just bring it back to focusing on the breath.
- Notice the intensity of your breathing – is it deep or shallow? Just observe, there is nothing to change or do. Just observe the in flow and out flow of your breath – just observe your breathing.
- Is it fast or slow? There is nothing to change – nothing is right or wrong.

Meditation 2   A different focus on your breathing

- Sit or lie in a comfortable position.
- Close your eyes and take a few relaxing breaths as in Meditation 1.
- Then begin to breathe normally and focus your attention on your breathing. Just observe your in breath and out breath; the rise and fall of your chest and abdomen as you breathe in and out. There is no need to try and change anything – just observe.

- If you find your attention wandering, just bring it back to your breathing – observing the in breath and the out breath.
- As you breathe in, say the word 'in' to yourself, and as you breathe out say the word 'out' to yourself.
- Prolong the enunciation of the word '**innnnnnnnnn**' so that it lasts for the entire 'in' breath.
- Prolong the enunciation of the word '**ouuuuuuuuuuuut**' so that it lasts for the entire 'out' breath. Just keep your focus on your breathing and if your mind wanders, keep bringing it back to your breathing.

Meditation 3   Colour exercise

Colour can have a profound effect on your mood, energy and well-being. We all know the uplifting effect that bright warm sunshine can have on us or, conversely, how a dark grey day can lower our spirits. Colour and light can make us feel better, more relaxed and happier.

Sit or lie down where you feel comfortable and relaxed, close your eyes and take a few relaxing breaths for a few moments. Breathe in to a count of 5 and breathe out slowly to a count of 9, and then begin to breathe normally. Now ....

- Imagine that you own a beautiful, big, circular, transparent shower.
- Inside this shower is a small panel containing three buttons.
- One button is marked 'calming blue light'; the next one 'sunshine cheer'; and the third one 'healing white light'.
- You can choose your desired colour by pressing the appropriate button. The whole shower area will become infused with your chosen colour. Also, the water-spray from the shower itself will take on your chosen colour.

- Imagine walking into your shower now and selecting the calming blue light.
- You are now standing in swirling calming blue light with calming blue water from the shower washing over your body.
- Feel the soothing caress and comfort of the warm blue water against your skin.
- As you breathe in, you inhale this relaxing calming blue light through the top of your head and imagine the blue calming light working its way all around your body, loosening blocks of stress and tension.

- You begin to feel the tension in your body slowly ebbing away with the water. You feel relaxed and great.

If you are doing this exercise in the daytime and need a bit more sunshine and joy in your life, switch on your sunshine button and bask in the shower of sunshine cheer.

If you feel over-wrought, you can use your healing white light.

Important reminder No. 1
Meditation can bring immediate calm to you.

Important reminder No. 2
Meditation can relieve your overall stress levels if you practise daily.

Resource 6
Anchor Yourself To Confidence & Good Feelings Using NLP

About NLP (neuro-linguistic programming) anchors

An anchor is a link or association we make between a certain sensory trigger and a specific feeling or state of mind. Anchors connect us to our memories, feelings and sensations.

An NLP anchor refers to the state of mind you want to create, for example, more confidence.

The trigger can be a sensory stimulus, for example, sound, touch hearing, taste or smell.

NLP anchoring gives you a quick and easy way to gain access to helpful emotions and resourceful states of mind on demand.

Ivan Pavlov, a Russian scientist, conditioned his dogs to salivate in response to a particular stimulus. The stimulus he used was the ringing of a bell. The dogs came to associate the ringing of the bell with food and salivated as a conditioned reflex. NLP anchoring is based on the same principle and works in the same way.

NLP anchors involve our senses and sensations

NLP anchors are composed of particular words, sounds, images, smells, tastes and sensations, such as physical touch. We don't need to involve all our senses to create an anchor. A physical touch combined with a word or two makes a good strong anchor.

Anchors provide *associations to memories and feelings* and are part of our daily lives. For example, a particular smell of fresh baked bread may evoke feelings of happiness in us because we associate it with happy childhood times. A particular tone of voice may evoke anxiety in us because of past negative associations. A certain song may evoke a romantic or nostalgic mood in us.

How you can create an NLP anchor

- You can create an NLP anchor by associating a unique trigger – such as a touch or words – with a certain positive emotion or state of mind – such as confidence or calmness.
- If you imaginatively relive an experience when, for example, you felt confident or calm, you can anchor yourself to these confident or calm feelings by using a particular stimulus, such as a particular touch or sound. Through repetition, that confident or calm state will be associated with the anchor you have created.
- Later, when you use the anchor, you will re-experience that confident or calm feeling.
- The more often you do this, the stronger the association, and the more effective the anchor becomes.

An exercise to create an anchor for confidence.

This same format can be applied to any positive emotion or state of mind you want to create. For example: more motivation, more relaxation.

Set aside 10–15 minutes when you won't be disturbed and make yourself comfortable, either sitting or lying down. Do a few minutes' relaxing breathing.

Exercise – NLP anchor – get confidence on tap

Tap into instant confidence

1 Call to mind a specific memory with strong feelings attached to it – when you truly felt super-confident and good about yourself. It might be, for example, when you passed your driving test, or an exam, learned to ride a bike, gave a great presentation, got the job you wanted, did well at something, or when the woman or man of your dreams agreed to go out with you!

2 Relive this experience again in your imagination as if you were actually there in it now, living it. See this experience in great detail through your own eyes, seeing again what you saw then, hearing again what you heard and feeling again what you felt – those good confident feelings – that put a big confident smile on your face. Soak in those strong feelings of confidence and self-belief.

3 Make the picture much bigger, bolder, brighter, more vibrant and colourful. Note if there are any sounds or smells involved. Identify what it is you are feeling and thinking that makes you feel so good and confident.

4 Intensify those good feelings. Do you feel these good feelings anywhere in your body? How are you standing? Looking? Notice just how confident you feel – if other people were there congratulating you, put them in the picture – and so see and hear them congratulating you and smiling and laughing with you.

5 **This is the important step.** When you are experiencing those great feelings most intensely, create your unique anchor. Press your right thumb into the centre of your left palm as if you were pressing a button there, while saying the words 'super-confidence' (hold for about 10 seconds).

6 **Now you take another very important step.** When you feel that confident state just starting to wane, release your Anchor and bring yourself into a neutral state of mind. Do this by thinking of something neutral or counting to 10.

7 **Trigger your anchor a few more times**
By triggering your Anchor, you are associating this particular pressure of your right thumb in the centre of your left palm with a strong feeling of confidence.

Now go through this confident memory by repeating steps 2, 3, 4, 5 and 6 and feel the great confident feelings again.

Do it at least five more times while using your anchor, pressing your right thumb into the centre of your left palm as if you were pressing a button there while saying the words 'super-confidence' (hold each time for about 10 seconds).

This will really lock in these good confident feelings.

You will know you have done this exercise enough times when all you need to do to experience confidence is to press your right thumb into the centre of your left palm there while saying the words 'super-confidence' (hold for about 10 seconds).

Repetition is the key to creating strong anchors.

You need to use your anchor regularly to create a conditioned response and increase the strength of your anchor.

If you want to set up more than one anchor, keep a note to remind yourself of which unique trigger you will use for each positive emotional state of mind you want to create (otherwise they won't work).

You can have several anchors on the go at any time.

Resource 7
Reduce Your Worries & Fears Using NLP

NLP exercise for reducing worries and fears

This is a very simple, powerful exercise that will enable you to reduce your fears or worries about a particular stressful situation in your life, or a certain person, or something that you are anxiously anticipating.

Relax first – sit down comfortably and close your eyes.

- Bring to mind a situation that you are anxious about.
- Notice what picture or scenario comes into your mind when you think about this situation.
- Imagine this picture or scenario on a big cinema screen in front of you, as if you were seeing it in a film. How big is your picture?
- Watch this film carefully, registering every detail and taking good note of what you can see, hear and feel.
- Is your film in colour or black and white? What exactly is happening in the film? Are there people? Can you hear any sounds or voices in the scene?
- Are people talking in it and, if so, what are they saying? What do their voices sound like – harsh, loud, accusing, or what?
- What do the people look like and what are they wearing? What expressions are on their faces?

- Take in every detail.
- Note what you are thinking and feeling as you look at the picture – anxious, worried and so on.

Now start changing the picture.

- Shrink the scene down to a smaller size.
- Drain the colour out of it. Make it dimmer, faded and blurred.
- Push the image further away from you into the distance.
- If there is a voice, make it squeaky, muffled, far away and indistinct.
- Change the speed of the voice, by making it very, very slow.
- Turn down the volume until the voice is barely audible, then turn it down all the way.

- **Now notice how you are feeling – less worried and fearful?**

Run through the above steps again several times very quickly which will further allay your anxiety.

Resource 8
Quick Stress-Busting Reminders

It's your life, look after yourself!

> Remember: taking control of your stress means taking good care of yourself on a daily basis.

1   **Breathe, breathe, and breathe!**
    When you half-breathe you half-live! It is the simplest and yet the most effective way to relieve your stress. You may need to learn how to breathe better and you need to remember to do your relaxing breathing frequently.

2   **Keep your blood sugar balanced!**
    During times of stress one of the most important things you can do is to look after your body in the best possible way. Stress affects your blood-sugar levels. By keeping blood-sugar levels in check, this will help reduce your stress. If you eat really well and regularly, you will immediately feel better.

    Always eat breakfast, lunch and dinner and include a few snacks throughout your day. Eat a diet rich in whole grains, pulses, nuts, seeds and eggs, with plenty of fresh fruit and vegetables. Include some protein in each meal and ensure that you eat some oily fish at least three times a week. Try to limit sugar, fat and processed foods. Sit down while eating, relax and give thanks for the food you are eating. Enjoy it to the full, knowing that you are showing your body the love and respect it deserves.

3   **Keep hydrated**
Really try to drink more water – at least eight glasses throughout the day.

4   **Sleep well**
Try to go to bed and get up at regular times every day and it will help you establish a better sleep pattern. Ensure that you get 7–8 hours a night. Your immune system and body need this time to recover, particularly when you are stressed.

Avoid any stimulating food or drink at bedtime – perhaps try some calming tea like valerian or chamomile. Do your 'Peaceful Haven' relaxing exercise or something similarly relaxing every day.

5   **Release body tension**
Remember your body tension-releasing exercises. Maintain good posture – it will help your mood and your breathing pattern.

6   **Get some exercise and fresh air**
Walk in the fresh air, in sunshine or in rain, for at least 15–20 minutes every day. Not only will it lift your mood but it will discharge some of your stress, keep you trimmer, fitter and healthier and often give you a different perspective on things.

Taking regular exercise will give you more energy and a sense of well-being.

7   **Lighten up yourself!**
Try not to take things too seriously, including yourself and others. Share a laugh with someone or watch or listen to a funny programme. Laughter can relieve stress and bring relaxing hormones into your blood.

8   **A problem shared is a problem halved**
Share a problem with someone you know you can trust. It can relieve some of your stress.

9   **Do something nice every day for yourself!**
Treat yourself and do something nice and special for yourself every day. Have a special relaxing bath, or a nice foot soak, listen to your favourite music, watch a favourite programme, cook something special for yourself or share it with a friend.

10 **Give your mind a break!**
Have a good novel on the go, or something else you like to read, and treat yourself to a short read of at least half an hour every day. This can help take you out of yourself and away from your everyday stresses and it is something you can enjoy.

Take a bit of time to do nothing every day. Just be yourself – sit and daydream or watch the birds.

If you can, do a bit of gardening or something creative like drawing or take up a creative interest.

11 **Remember, remember the good things you have**
Remember to appreciate yourself and others, the little and big things you have in your life, and give thanks for what you have.

12 **Kindness and generosity to yourself and others**
These go a long way towards making you happier and more content.

13 **Create your own happy hormones**
Dwelling on any beautiful or happy experience in your life, or a happy fantasy, imagining a beautiful scenic place, like the top of a lovely mountain or a tropical island – even for a few moments – can bring cheering hormones into your blood and change negative feelings.

14 **Let your heart heal you**
Use the great heart changing exercises in the HeartMath section in Chapter 16.

15 **Take courage, be brave and face up to your problems and dilemmas**
Taking action to deal with anything in life that stresses you, resolving your problems and standing up for yourself are great steps forward in your emotional development.

Remember, if you have difficulty dealing with any aspect of your life and feel held back, it is courageous and brave to seek professional help.

We would strongly advise this.

We are all human, we all suffer and we all need help at times.

Maggie and Sylvia send best wishes and kind regards and wish for you the good things in life you truly deserve.

Lightning Source UK Ltd.
Milton Keynes UK
UKOW031207180612

194621UK00002B/22/P